T0131685

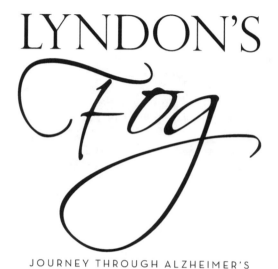

LYNDON'S Fog

JOURNEY THROUGH ALZHEIMER'S

CAROLYN BAGNALL

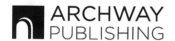

ARCHWAY
PUBLISHING

Archway Publishing books may be ordered through booksellers or by contacting:

Archway Publishing
1663 Liberty Drive
Bloomington, IN 47403
www.archwaypublishing.com
844-669-3957

Interior Graphics/Art Credit: Carolyn Bagnall

ISBN: 978-1-6657-3114-0 (sc)
ISBN: 978-1-6657-3113-3 (hc)
ISBN: 978-1-6657-3379-3 (e)

Library of Congress Control Number: 2022919669

Print information available on the last page.

Archway Publishing rev. date: 03/13/2023

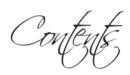

Contents

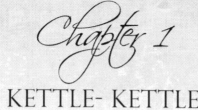

KETTLE- KETTLE

"If I say the words 'kettle, kettle' that is your clue that I'm telling you that you have Alzheimer's, and you are to cooperate with me," I sigh as I speak to my eldest brother, David, over the phone. He is a thousand miles away from the heat of the situation, Dad's failing mental status and incoming fog. "You do know it's hereditary and with me being the youngest, I might have to take care of you if you get it," I say half joking half serious.

"Ok, kettle, kettle," he repeats. "I've got it. Now what about a kettle?" he mocks trying to make light of the circumstances.

"You have no idea of what Mark and I are going through here," I say flatly somewhat annoyed. Mark, my other brother, is living with Dad, yet with Mark's full-time day job, the daily 'dropping-in' every morning will become my new career.

I know in my heart that David cares about Dad, but he is not able to really help carry this load. Every member of the family though will enter the emotional paper shredder and eventually, we will all come through with torn hearts.

I now know why I picked the words 'kettle-kettle' to be the code phrase for Alzheimer's. I stood in the home section of the department store looking for a Christmas present for my dad and my eyes fell upon an electric kettle with a safety shut off feature. He loves tea. He and his second wife had teatime throughout the day. In fact, it had become increasing impossible for Dad to complete any project because the prim little English woman would crack open the side screen door and call, "Lyndon, it's teatime." He would shuffle up the side porch stairs in his hunter green work pants and stained blackened work boots to sip English tea and dip biscuits. Stopping work projects is like turning off all the lights in an old cathedral. If one succeeded, one does not really want to go back and turn them all back on when tea break is finished. Even after my stepmother's death the tradition continues. Work and putter until you need an excuse to quit. Teatime is the perfect excuse. Concentrating on puttering projects became increasingly confusing and often he would take a break, sit, and doze off. On more than one occasion, a high-pitched whistling sound woke my napping father who had started to make tea but settled into his comfortable wingback chair forgetting the kettle on the stove. The charred almost bottomless stove-top kettle needed replacing because the risk of fire was too great. I picked it up, that brand-new electric kettle with a safety shut off feature and placed it in my cart. This was the first Alzheimer's gift I purchased before I knew he had the disease.

As he opened the gift that Christmas Day, I smiled, knowing I have done my part to protect my dad from serious injury. This gift would help him to continue living independently in his home. He unwrapped the gift and placed the kettle on the nearby marbled coffee table. The refracted rays of the winter sun through the window highlighted the light pink skin on his neck where he had been seriously burned many years before while doing his job as a city bus driver.

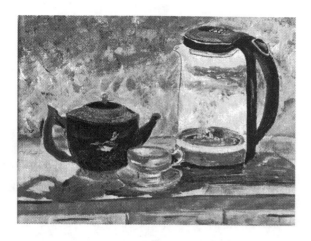

The early morning sun kissed the newly built homes in the northwest London community as Father drove his bus through the quiet neighborhood. Something was wrong. He pulled the London city bus over as steam poured out. He knew, as a driver, he should call it in and wait for a new bus or for the company to send out a man to fix this one. In that moment he decided that maybe it was something small which he could remedy on his own. The thought of the university students who needed to be at their early morning labs and the factory workers whose shifts would begin shortly plagued him. They would be waiting at their respective bus stops for him. Some of the passengers loved to joke with him, some were quiet, but he kindly welcomed each, on his run-down city bus as if they were entering a wedding limo and it was going to be the best day of their life.

"I'll just open the cover and let the bus radiator cool down," he muttered to himself as he started turning the lid. With the speed of a baseball leaving a pitcher's hand and with the force of a fire hydrant uncapped, boiling hot water gushed out in a violent stream toward my father. In a split second the horizontal steaming geyser from a lake of hell itself, narrowly missed his face, but its full fury struck his neck and back as he turned. The air on the quiet street was punctuated with a piercing hyena yelping sound as my father ran like a wounded animal to the front door of a house on a perfectly manicured lawn. Banging with desperate fists, yelling and ringing the bell, he screamed for help.

Terrified and bewildered the woman cautiously opened the door to see a middle-aged man stripping off his uniform hollering, "Get me water!" In horror she gripped the doorknob and took in the whole scene—the raw flesh of a man peeling off, and behind him was a bus steaming in the morning light as the geyser slowed from the bus. "Water, get me cold water," he whimpered, slumping over.

Shaken into action, she half pulled, half dragged the man to her shower. Clothes, puddles, and skin littered the route. Through his renewed screaming and moaning she yanked on the elephant shower head, dousing him in cold water. With his strength gone, father fell against the translucent door as his body collapsed to the floor. Thud!

"Come fast!" she screamed as she repeated her address to the 911 operator. Barely conscious and face down, half naked on the tiled glistening floor with stinging droplets pelting him, his mind reeled.

I knew that he often asked people if they were ready to meet the Lord. Some had listened while others had not. His encounter with a hellish hot stream of water renewed his mission in life to tell others about a literal Hell. It was horrible and he didn't want anyone to suffer. His Saviour had suffered so they could escape torment and live eternally in heaven.

Over the next few weeks, they grafted on pig skin. They wrapped him like a mummy in a horror movie. Once they had forgotten him in a salt bath leaving him to crawl naked back to his hospital room. He healed and I am sure every nurse and attendant heard about his Jesus. He survived.

With dementia however, the body seems fine, but the mind is slowly short circuiting. It is burning out and the charred remains of each compartment of the brain turns to ash. First one's short-term memory goes. *Did I leave the kettle on?* Next, one's emotional stability is fractured; one's personality changes. One's filter of appropriateness blazes into wild colours. Then long-term memories burn into oblivion, and finally bodily functions deteriorate. Death often comes from a lodged piece of food or a heart forgetting to pound. The gray spaghetti mind is slowly burning on the stove, and everyone knows it but the person himself.

Chapter 2

I DIDN'T DO THAT

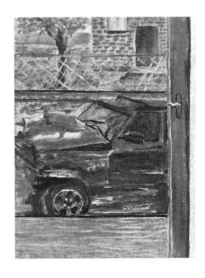

Cement sidewalks have predictable cut lines every two and a half feet, but as my dad's 'concrete' mind deteriorates, the regular paths of thought develop cracks and its corners crumble. Weeds of confusion protrude through every crevice making it impossible to travel coherently in the here and now.

"Dad, what happened to the car?" I gasp while sitting at the kitchen table looking through the back screen door at the crushed

Cherokee Jeep. The vehicle resembled a smashed Halloween pumpkin.

"Oh, that little dent. I just bumped a guideline. You know, those yellow wires that run up to the telephone pole," he gestures with an upward hand movement. "The lady on the other side would have hit me head-on so I swerved to avoid an accident."

"Some bump," I sigh as my eyes scan the mangled grill and follow the folded front end up to the windshield. "What did the police officer say?" I queried.

My dad crosses the kitchen floor and pours old tea into his already full cup stopping only when it begins to overflow onto the counter.

Leaning in, my brother whispers, "Some witnesses said that he was avoiding an accident while another witness said that he just turned and drove straight for the pole, but luckily smacked into the wire first to lessen the impact."

Not sure what to do with an overflowing cup of tea, my dad answers, "Well, I don't know exactly what the police officer said, something about owing money to the city for damages and that I was lucky he wasn't giving me a careless driving charge." Slightly louder and becoming agitated he continues, "I did not cause any damage, and I have no intention of paying that bill. It's a lucky thing I did what I did, or there would have been a real accident!"

I slump into the chair not knowing how to proceed. This man was morphing into someone whose reality was flickering, and by the end of the week he would argue that he hadn't hit anything at all. In later months he began to ask, "Who smashed up my car?"

The sun streamed through the same cloudy glass screen door and in my mind I see a smashed bike laying on the cement behind the 1975 station wagon. The door flew open, "Carolyn, you'd better come here now."

I hardly ever recall hearing that tone in my father's voice because rarely did he ever raise his voice or show annoyance with us kids. I plopped down the fistful of monopoly money, grabbed the railing taking two steps at a time to reach the top stair. My neighbourhood friend stood at the bottom of the stairs waiting.

"No, you need to see this too", my father motioned to my friend to join us.

Pushing through the door we both stopped, stood, and stared. My shiny blue bike with the silver bell stood upright on the kickstand to the left of the driveway near the house just where Melinda had left it.

That sticky afternoon my friend, Melinda, and I had decided to switch bikes to play cops and robbers. My blue bike had been designated as the cop bike and her worn out banana-seat golden bike would be the robber bike. We both drove wildly up and down the sidewalk until we were overcome by the heat. Melinda gave up the chase and parked my bike up near the house while I discarded her bike behind our green and brown station wagon in the driveway.

"Race you to the house for a popsicle!" I hollered with a head start toward the house. We burst through the door—bikes forgotten.

My father cleared his throat bringing us back.

"But Father, I didn't know you were going out. I just put Melinda's bicycle down." I couldn't continue as I stared at the twisted wheel of her bike which looked like modern metal art.

"Since you put your friend's bike behind the car where I couldn't see it when I tried to back out . . ." he left the sentence to finish itself with a gesture toward the smashed bike. "What do you think we should do?" he asked looking at me.

I shrugged my shoulders knowing, but not knowing, what he would suggest. "Replace it?" I stammered.

My heart sank. I didn't have any way to earn money and her bike was old. My mind raced rationalizing the consequences. The firm lines on my father's face were dissipating as if he could read my thoughts.

"Melinda," he turned and addressed my friend, "I am sorry I ran over your bike, and I realize that it wasn't your fault since Carolyn left it there. So, if your parents think this would be fair, Carolyn's new bike will be yours."

I felt as though I was a snail on a sidewalk crunched under a bike tire, embarrassed, angry, and humiliated; but I knew my father was right. I had put the bike there. It was my fault and the only way to make it right was to give her my new bike. Together we picked up the twisted metal and after setting it aside, I gently pushed the kickstand down and wheeled my sparkling aqua-marine blue bike toward my friend and whispered, "Sorry".

She was uncomfortable too, but with her hands on the white tinsel handlebars she began slowly to walk toward her home. I turned and my wet tears soaked my father's shirt. Patting my sweaty fine curls, he cooed, "It's ok. It was the right thing to do. Now run along and explain it to her parents."

The right thing to do is often taught to us by our parents and their code of ethics, wherever they have learned it. For our family the code was the Bible. For me that day, I needed to give her my bike for restitution due to my carelessness. However, now in this new reality of dementia, responsibility and truth-telling are flipped on their head.

No one in the family is allowed to remove the smashed vehicle to make room. It is as though the crushed metal Jeep is invisible and the accident never happened, and no responsibility for its occurrence has been taken. It is a reminder that what is real may be right in front of us, but it isn't really seen. The gray-haired man I see now is not who I once beheld. This man's new ethical code does not match the father who taught me the right thing to do.

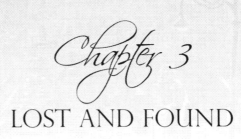

Chapter 3

LOST AND FOUND

M OST PEOPLE THINK OF DEMENTIA OR A LZHEIMER'S PATIENTS IN terms of those odd old people who wander off aimlessly lost. My father knew the city better than me. He knew the streets, the boulevards, and the cul-de-sacs like a migrating bird that knows its way across continents and oceans. He drove so many different bus routes over and over that it was etched into his mind like the carved path of a fast-flowing river. In London, Ontario, the Thames River threads its way through the forest city forcing city engineers to build bridges and design roads around it and he knew them all.

Eventually, my dad began to report," I couldn't find Dan and Kathy's house today so I went downtown and found my way home after some driving," or "I was so confused I couldn't find the store where Mark asked me to pick up the photos?"

On one Thursday afternoon my children tell Grampy, "Mom's not here," when he calls looking for me. "She is waiting at the library for you to pick her up." He has forgotten how to get there and by the time he gets back home he forgets why he went out.

On the downward slide, he begins to use the car to look for his dead wife; driving from place to place. She didn't want to accept her coming death and yet it came upon her failing body. He obviously hasn't accepted it or had forgotten it.

"She's out there!" he firmly claims. He first begins searching down the old streets where she'd lived as a widow before he had married her. "Why won't she just come home?" The question causes such pain in his soul.

"Carolyn, you must call all the nursing homes to find her. She has probably booked herself into one." The basic truth that she's dead which I try again and again to tell him only aggravates the situation. After a short reflection and an empty stare, he retorts, "You've got the wrong woman. I am talking about Irene. I'm going to the retirement home to look for her." He will never find her and looking only deepens his desire to find her.

On many mornings I suggest, "How about you drive over here, and we will go together?" I have laundry, dishes, and other plans, but this is becoming my new life—looking for a dead stepmother. It sounds like a new video game release. If I don't laugh at the craziness of it all, I will bawl and not be able to stop.

"Well, let's look for her," I say agreeing to the game. I will make this into an opportunity to check out the nursing home as a possible future home for my dad when the time comes. The lady at the home graciously walked us from room to room helping us look for a dead woman all the while showing my dad and I the neatly kept rooms available. He sits on one of the beds and in a lucid moment he asks, "So what's the price if I had to move in?"

After the lady responds, clouds of worry cloak his face as his mind begins again chasing the foggy thought. With his head in his cupped hands he whispers, "Where could she have gone?" I recognize the look of his stinging tears because I had briefly been the cause of similar tears in his eyes many years before. I returned home late but not lost.

"I am seven! Can't I go to the pool with James by myself, Mom?" I argued. Mom had spent every afternoon walking James and me to the park pool at the end of the street to swim. After a few hours of sitting and watching on the other side of the silver chain-linked fence, she would fold up her lawn chair when the closing whistle blew and walk us home.

"I will go straight to the pool and be home shortly after 4:30 when the pool closes," I continued to plead my case.

Reluctantly, she smoothed her hands on the fabric of her yellow polka-dotted dress. "Alright, but come straight home when the swim ends," she instructed. I'd be home I assured her.

James was the little boy who I had played with all summer. We had eaten chocolate whoppers from milk carton shaped boxes until we were almost sick in his small house. We rode bikes and climbed trees. We enjoyed our childhood summer freedom. I flung the towel over my shoulder determined to be a big girl now. James could not believe it when I knocked on his door and my mom wasn't on the sidewalk with her old, orange lawn chair in hand.

"Really? Your mom said we could go to the pool by ourselves?" he reached around the corner grabbing his towel. He had the funkiest, green frog swimsuit and brown flip flops. We skipped down the block singing. "Step on a crack and break your mother's back." We would never have sung that if my mother was walking with us. The cool aqua-blue pool was just about to open as the red suited lifeguards took their high seated places around it. We jumped off the diving board, somersaulted underwater and swam under each other's legs until we were exhausted.

"Let's leave a little early and take a different path home," James suggested. I trusted James. His wild blonde hair flew around even when it was drenched. With flip flops on and towels draped over our shoulders, we set out on an adventure. Of course, we'd be home by 4:30. Down Park Avenue we walked and talked and giggled. We made up new rhymes and played trains by tying our towels together and 'choo-chooed' as we turned unfamiliar street corners. James confidently told me that he knew where we were, and I never questioned it.

Suppertime had long passed. We had walked on streets that I had only driven on with my parents, but as promised, James finally got us back home. He waved and scooted into his tin roofed home, which had no cars in the driveway. But at my house the family car was blocked in by a police cruiser. My shadow covering two cracks on the sidewalk should have made me realize the lateness of the day. I slipped in the door knowing we had taken the long route home and that I was probably a little late, but I did not realize the gravity of the situation. My father's cupped hands held his drooped head. "I don't know where she could be."

"Who?" I asked cluelessly. The commotion was all about me. Joy, fear, anger, and surprise crossed my parents faces almost simultaneously as they immediately jumped off the couch to hug me. Tears streamed down my mother's face as she scooped me up. I looked over her shoulder past my father and saw the clock. I was in trouble! It was way past my bedtime! Yet the feared consequences never came. I had disobeyed. I had scared my parents half to death, and my mother's orange lawn chair returned as a permanent fixture every afternoon outside the gated park pool for the rest of the summer.

Lost is awful if you know and odd if you are unaware but excruciating for the people awaiting your return. With Alzheimer's you never return mentally though physically you may wander back home.

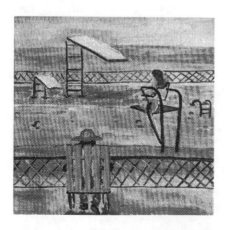

Chapter 4

UNCONTROLLABLE

Two-year-olds throw tantrums; teenagers fume and slam doors. Sadly, seniors with dementia do both. As a young man, my father had the odd altercation growing up in the late 1940's. I heard stories of his threatening methods to get his money back when he loaned it out. He'd always recall these times shaking his head as if to lose the memory from his mind and then he would paraphrase "But that was before I became a new creation in Christ, old things have passed away and all things become new."[1]

I was the third child of a first-generation born-again believer and my father was anything but violent. His kindness towards my mother was demonstrated through cooking meals when she worked afternoons, scrubbing the kitchen floor when he saw she was too busy and it needed cleaning, and even vacuuming the rugs throughout the house to try out one of the new Electrolux models he would be selling on the weekend. His gentleness and kindness extended to us kids as well. He was not a push over parent, but he was the parent

---

[1]   2 Corinthians 5:17 King James Version

you'd ask if you wanted a 'yes' answer. Violence, which permeates some homes, was never present in ours.

I'm going out to look for Irene!" I heard a jingle as my dad pulled the keys off the rack. My stepmother, Irene, his second wife, had succumbed four years earlier to the havoc-wreaking disease of cancer just as my mother had fifteen years before that.

"No, we've talked about this, you can't drive at night," my brother states, in a steady but firm voice.

The air is tense. "Yes, I am!" boomed the retort. The words tumbled out from the lips of a failing eighty-year-old much like a determined teenager attempting to take the car for a spin.

"No!" Mark pushed away from the downstairs computer desk, ran up the stairs, and faced off with the man. My brother had become a wonderful young man, but as a teen, he was a tornado waiting for a place to touch down. This clash had reversed; my brother, 'the parent', tried to make our dad, 'the teen', drop the keys into his open hand. I watched the seen unfold in slow motion.

With a fistful of keys dad raised his clenched hand and hollered, "This is my house. I'll go and come when I want. I am going out to find Irene!" We knew his search was fruitless. I could see his glazed look was not one of a docile half-sleeping kitten, but one of a tiger in a cage enraged by kids poking at it with sticks.

Raising the anti, Mark declared war, "No Dad, you cannot GO!!" and tried to pry the keys from his fist.

The landing was small where both men squared-off. In my mind I heard the popping sound of fireworks before the light show. Leaping up the stairs I thrust myself between them.

"Dad," I pleaded, "You can't go out." Mark stepped back knowing his emotions equaled an igniting rocket.

I would take the blows if I had to. This was foreign ground for me to stand between such raw anger. Looking into my dad's clouded eyes was almost like seeing a monster and a frightened child all tangled up. I did not recognize him. The fog thickened. I did not face Mark because at that moment I realized all the frustration and stress of several months of constant evening and weekend caregiving had reached his fists. The initial swell and wave of emotion swept over the three of us, but as I reached for the keys slowly, thinking I had diffused the situation, the second wave came.

"Move your car, Carolyn" he growled, "or I'll drive right over it!" I became a child at 47. I obediently reached for my keys and held my other hand up to keep my brother at bay.

How could tiny bits of protein travel within the human brain and destroy a stable man's emotions creating this lack of self-control. Many years before my father had experienced the violent emotional outburst of another elderly gentleman.

My father sold Electrolux as a part time job, but his love and primary job was driving a city bus. As a child, I ran around the house with his bus cap and coat on pretending to careen around the corners of our living room and kitchen. On that morning I was no longer a child, but a university student. Split shifts for bus drivers were common and my father had finished the first part of his shift from 5 am to 9 am. He pulled his bus into a stop in the core of downtown London. Into the heavy morning fog, he stepped down into the street. With his lunch pail in hand he was ready to board another bus home when his smile morphed into a gasp.

The knife penetrated with each stab; the repeated slicing and slashing continued to puncture his neck and back. Blood flew in every direction. The half-crazed attacker struck my father from behind relentlessly. Some people gawked. Some people parted. Some people ran. Only one brave black woman from a war-torn African country acted. She clobbered the aggressor from behind and in a moment of surprise the tide turned. Police officers on the downtown beat subdued the knife waving, demented man. My father fell to the ground covered in his own blood. Moments later my brother received a call.

"Son, we have a man down here. It's your father. He has been stabbed. Come to the corner of Richmond and Dufferin Street." These staccato sentences ignited my brother into action. Mark slammed down the phone, grabbed the keys, and darted in and out of traffic like a rabbit on the run through brambles. Squealing tires ceased. He shoved through the crowd yelling, "That's my father!"

The pool of blood looked like an TV crime scene with the one officer slapping handcuffs on the deranged man on the ground. Thinking his father was dead, and this man lay in his father's blood, justice needed to be meted out now. My brother reacted. He dove towards the man, but the man in blue clamped his hand on Mark's shoulder to intervene. He calmed him and reasoned with him. The officer reassured Mark that his father would live.

Our father recovered from his numerous stab wounds. But what of the mentally challenged old man? He was found guilty but served no jail time. They put him in an institution for the mentally unstable for a short time.

Unstable, uncontrolled, negative aggression—had I just witnessed those same emotions in my own dad because of a disease, Alzheimer's? My father from the past had forgiven the wild man who attacked him and who now roams in the streets free. I would forgive my dad as I heard the tires squeal and he drove away searching for a dead woman whom he believed was alive and needed to be found.

- ❋ -

CAROLYN BAGNALL

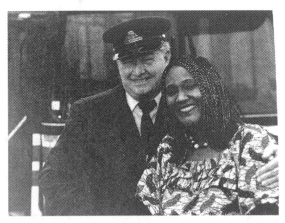

PHOTO- Reader's Digest July 1998 Heroes for Today

Chapter 5

IT IS THE TIME OF YOUR LIFE

IN THE PAST, THE PHRASE A 'BROKEN RECORD' WOULD BE understood, but in my generation, there is no equivalent phrase to describe a scratched CD. I sang as the words blared through my car speakers. *"You are the Dancing Queen, young and sweet, only seventeen."* I continued in rhythm to the words *"You can dance, you can jive, having the time of your life,"* time of your life, time of your life, time of your life,'[2]

"AHH! My ABBA CD! It is scratched!" Yanking the CD out, I rub the silver magic disc of music on the soft green fabric of my favourite shirt as the rain begins to plop on the windshield. Similarly, my dad is stuck in the 'time of his life'. Old memories are repeated in a stuck old 'broken record' way. I remember telling Mark, "It can't be that bad. What's the big deal if he repeats a question or a story?"

However, I begin to see for myself when I spend more time with him. One evening while I am visiting, Mark informs Dad, "I'm going to the store. I'll be right back."

"Where are you going?"

"The store, we need groceries," Mark states again.

---

[2]   ABBA Dancing Queen August 15, 1976, music

Dad looks at Mark sliding his coat on, and as if there had been no prior conversation, he initiates a new one, "Where are you going?"

Slightly annoyed, he responds civilly, "To the store, to get the milk we need, Dad."

Dad looks, processes, and then loses the information. The conversation is like a wave washing over the shore. "Mark, where are you going?"

Mark grabs the keys. Ignoring the question, he looks over in my direction and mouths the words silently, "Now, do you see what I go through?"

Dad turns to me and speaks in a frustrated tone, "He never tells me where he is going. He just takes off."

The repetitious conversations can be trying. However, when the recollection of the memories changes and false new realities are etched deeper into the mind of someone losing their mind, you begin to question your own sanity. Before dementia dragged its debilitating fingers into Dad's brain, he would walk into stores and speak to anyone who would engage in conversation. The standard answer he gave when someone asked how he was doing, was, "I'm not doing bad for a man who has lost two wives." I would just keep shopping as they continued talking but one day the painful truth of the death of his wives changed.

"Where's Irene? She must have left me and hasn't come home." Dad announces this new 'truth' out of the blue.

She had often travelled during their marriage and visited her sister in British Columbia, or her niece near Ottawa or gone for long walks by herself. While my father and his first wife, (my mother), had done everything together, Irene was her own person and having been widowed before she'd married father, she wasn't about to be smothered by some man who wanted to know about her whereabouts 24/7. This simple difference by both parties created some challenges for them as a senior couple going to the altar. Yet this twist—this new reality—which he created no one could have foreseen. His new purpose in life became searching for Irene like a child looking for Waldo in a picture book. I had been visiting every morning now as part of my routine, but unbeknownst to me, Dad would head out in his car many afternoons investigating leads of her whereabouts. My brother and I knew he often took the car out right after dinner for a drive 'to find her'. However, things were about to get interesting.

"Hello, are you Lyndon MacBain's son?" the man dressed in uniform queried. "We've had a complaint from a resident on Park Avenue regarding your dad knocking at their door this evening looking for his wife."

Things were out of hand. He drove to nursing homes and frequented antique stores looking for her. Because he sounded so sane, so concerned, many thought that his wife was the one that had dementia and must be lost. The daily drives, the intermittent police check-ins, and this constant obsession was about to bring my brother to his breaking point.

When in university, I took pride in staying up all night before exams or for assignments, but my brother treasured his sleep, and he was the one living with Dad now. Many nights, Dad would wake up yelling from nightmares, pace the floor, and then make tea. All this commotion would wake up Mark, who lived downstairs and needed his sleep to work the next day. Mark, groggy and blurry eyed, would come up the stairs and attempt to light the way for this troubled ship in a fog to come to harbour, to get Dad back to bed so they could both get some more sleep.

If it was only occasionally, he could have handled it, but the regularity of the nightly shenanigans was exhausting. Mark was at the end of his rope. His voice was desperate when he called early that morning, "I'm through, Carolyn! He will have to go into a home. I cannot be up half the night with him. Something has got to change. He is crazy about finding Irene and roams the house at night like a racoon rummaging through garbage."

My mind reeled. Overall, he wasn't too difficult but, on this issue, he'd jumped overboard and there was no way to drag him back onto the ship of truth. The truth for him was foggy. We knew she was dead yet announcing that quietly or in strong terms only made his commitment to this imagined reality stronger. I would have to break the tether and lie.

Chapter 6

LYING FOR TRUTH

THIS WAS GOING TO BE THE LARGEST CONCOCTED LIE I COULD think of. I would fill it with emotions so dramatic that he would have to come to the truth; Irene was dead. The music was about to play, *"the time of your life, see that girl, watch that scene digging the Dancing Queen."*[3] I wasn't a dancer, but I was going to have to be the best actress in my one debut, <u>Finding Nemo</u> (Irene) or my father would be lost at sea. I wrestled with my conscience and the ethical decision to lie. In classes on dementia, they tell you to 'play along' with their reality—LIE. I had committed then that I would not do that, but that was in the past. Thus far I had been able to nod my head instead of constantly disagreeing with him, but I had not outright lied. Things were different now; I began to rationalize. David in the Bible feigned madness to save his life. Christians and other concerned citizens hid Jews during WWII, living lives of deceit to save them. I know of present-day missionaries who lie to sneak Bibles into forbidden lands. This cause isn't as noble or grand but my love for Dad ran like veins of gold under a rock. Lying might set the dynamite charges and things might explode if he were to uncover the plot. He might never trust me again, or maybe I would

---

3   ABBA Dancing Queen August 15, 1976, music

travel this morally sketchy road only to have this man completely forget the drama the next day, but I plunged on.

I called my Christian friends to pray. I don't know if I called them out of a guilty conscience or a desire for success. I chose to lie to get to the truth and to stop the incessant driving and to bring closure to his troubled mind. I walked into his house with a pace like molasses from a carton that morning. The black sticky lie would have to be poured on thick.

"Dad," I whimper, "I need to tell you something. You'd better sit down. It's about Irene."

"Did you find her?" he asks with full attention.

"No, I got a call," I take a shallow breath and continue, "from an officer in Ottawa. Irene escaped from the nursing home and travelled on this past long weekend without identification and she . . ." I pause for effect and wipe the corner of my eye, "she had a heart attack on the train." I wait to see if anything is being understood in his weary mind. "I can't believe she's dead," I continue, not sure if he is even following the tale I am spinning. Glancing up with fake tears in my eyes, I see fear and pain beginning to emerge on his face. I feel like a butcher, looking the cow in the eye while I bring down the knife. "They already buried her and I . . ." sniffing slightly, "think we have to find out if its true."

My mother always told me how one lie leads to another and then another. I had never truly experienced the magnitude of this truth until today.

"Well, why didn't they call me after they figured out who she was?"

"You were sleeping this morning (that part was true), and you must not have heard the phone," (that part was a lie).

"They couldn't bury her without notifying me first," he struggled to put the pieces together.

Trying to stop the barrage of questions and the lying cycle, I countered, "Let's go to the cemetery to see if she's been buried in London."

I know she is there because after her battle with cancer, she died in the winter, and we buried her in the spring at Forest Lawn in 2010. Anytime my brother or I tried to take him to see her gravestone, he had refused and argued that he was talking about a different woman than we were, and that we were the ones mixed up. I drive Dad to the well-manicured cemetery, and we slowly walk toward the office. I try to arrive first to ask the lady to play along before he pushes through the double doors behind me.

"We have been informed that Irene MacBain has died on a train, and we think she was buried here. This is her husband. We want to verify her death." The lady plays along but cannot find any record of Irene MacBain. I begin to think I am crazy. I know I could throw a baseball from the porch of the building, and it would land on her plot. The receptionist, however, suggests that we go home and call the funeral home to find out where we thought the police may have sent the body for burial. Now she was lying. Where was the body? "*What is wrong with her records?*" I think to myself.

"*Oh, the tangled web, we weave*"[4] I recall from a line in Walter Scott's poem. I call the funeral home, trying my best to remember which funeral home we had used four years ago. The woman assured me that indeed she was buried at the Forest Lawn Cemetery. When my dad left to walk across the kitchen to make a cup of tea, I whisper why I was doing this into the receiver and explain the whole sordid tale in muffled tones. She then offers to send out a death certificate asking if that would help. She explains to me that she could 'white out' the death date and write in a current death date to give validity to my story. As Dad approaches, I repeat loudly, "Oh that would be good if you could send us a death certificate." Dad returns to the kitchen chair with his piping hot tea.

---

[4]   Sir Walter Scott, poem Marmion 1808.

Doubt was shifting to belief like clouds promising rain, but just like the weather, one never knows for sure. I knew he would need more. I step outside, pretending to get something out of the van and call my friend to see if her husband would phone the house posing as the responder on site when the train tragedy occurred. Upon returning into the house, the phone is already ringing, jolting my father back from his 'tea' induced state.

"I am Chris, a person on site at the accident, and I am so sorry to inform you . . ." and as the story is retold my dad begins to interrogate the man.

"Why didn't you call me earlier? Are you sure it was my wife?" my dad is agitated.

The man on the other end answered all the questions. Dad hands me the phone and I return it to the cradled hook.

"It's really true," he chews the information as though he was trying to swallow bitter kale. "She's passed. I can hardly believe it," he utters barely audible.

"Well, let us go back out to the cemetery and see if the cemetery lady was misinformed." During the solemn quiet drive, I try to fathom why the woman could not find the record of her death the first time. My mind unravelled the mystery! The name engraved on the stone would have been her first husband's name.

"Irene Siegrist. Do you have a record for an Irene Siegrist buried here?" I announced proud to have solved the case of the dead but not buried. The woman scans the computer and smiles politely as she tells us where to go to see the grave site. Her eyes search my face probably wondering if I had thought of my explanation for the wrong date on the gravestone. I am ready, yet nervous. As I step outside, I begin scanning the ground for any natural object, I can use to cover the ending zero in the year '2010'. Casually I retie my shoes to retrieve a crumbled leaf from the ground. Would he really believe she is gone? The peaking sunshine mocks me as it glittered on the short well-kept grass as though it might undo all the deception.

I dropped the leaf and moved it discreetly with the toe of my shoe over the last zero in 2010.

"I can't believe it. It really must be true," I sniffle looking down at the gravestone.

He pauses, "No, she's not dead or her body isn't here." he flatly stated with defiance. He isn't looking at the date on the stone but at the ground. The grass is perfect. She wasn't buried here, or it would be all torn up.

What logic! What perfect detective senses! My mind goes into overdrive.

I had done so much work to get him to believe that she had died on the train and was buried here this past weekend. It is like planning for someone's surprise birthday and forgetting the cake. This was one detail I had not planned on.

"Let's go back in and ask her," I suggest as we walk away from the grave. The woman behind the elbow high counter tries to explain to dad that the sod could settle down quite well in two days, but that she would check the records again to be sure.

"Well maybe she was buried in Ottawa." I replied to the woman sounding defeated. "You do your research and call me on my cell," I comment, knowing that if Dad interrogates her further, things will get tricky.

Silently I drive him back home.

To remove a scratch from a CD you can use car wax and gently rub the solution on the etched groove. I had poured a bottle of lies on my father's warped etched memory. Would the 'search for Irene' groove be erased, and this new memory implanted? I leave him with his thoughts. The soap opera for today done. The air in the van hangs with the sound waves of lies. What I had done was atrocious! I feel like a criminal with the guilt of the lies weighing heavily on me.

"God, if this was not the way you wanted me to handle this, please erase this from his mind by morning, and I'll continue to help him with his search for Irene," I pray under my breath.

The next few days bring more lies to continue the cover story. He wants answers regarding the funeral costs, the will, the bank accounts, and her belongings. The snowball of lies causes an avalanche, but over the next few weeks, as we dig our way out from under the mountain of snow, there is a quiet serenity. The agitation which had controlled my dad decreases as I answer every question for many weeks. Each day now, I simply remind him of her death on the train to Ottawa and this new reality usually helps him skip over the scratched CD-like brain, but not always.

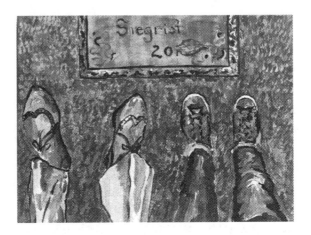

Chapter 7

LAYING ASIDE THE CHEF'S HAT

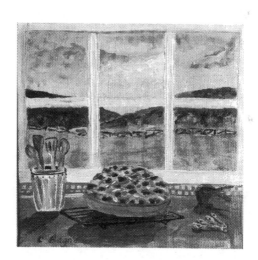

With dementia the losses may be small or large, but they are accumulative. If the losses an Alzheimer's patient experiences could be represented by clothing on a clothesline, that line would cross acres of farmland. With clothes pins in hand, I hang the chef's apron on the line of losses.

My brother thought that maybe our dad was lazy because he would make excuses for not preparing dinner. I knew laziness was not the reason because the father I knew did not have a lazy bone in him. He was a hard worker and always did what needed to be done.

"I don't think he can cook now," I whisper to my brother. He groans, having to make dinner again after a long day at work, while Dad sits at the kitchen table staring into his teacup as though it would reveal his fortune.

"I reminded him on my lunch break and left a note which told him to put the pork chops in the oven at 4:30, prepare the vegetables, and make a box cake. How hard can it be? He needs something to do when he's not out with you," Mark mutters.

"How hard is it, to make a box cake?" I think to myself as my brother's frustrated speech winds down.

"Well, first you must retrieve the mixer out from beneath the oak cupboard under the sink," I process with my sharp brain. This is not fair. I need to really try to imagine what it is like for him with little to no short-term memory. The conversation in his mind might look like this I conjecture.

Yes, I need the cake mix. Mark wants me to make a cake. Let's see, I need to make it in something. The mixer. . . now where is that mixer? I don't see it here, nor under there. What about up here? I can't find that . . . what am I looking for? Let me sit down and think. (Reads the note 'make cake') Ah yes, 'the mixer'. (15 minutes of rummaging and he finds the mixer.) Now put the cake mix in the bowl. Where are those blasted scissors to cut open the bag of cake mix? (He turns and sees a cup of tea) I think I will heat up this tea . . .

. . . (opening the microwave, he notices . . .) The scissors? What are they doing in the microwave? I'll just put them on the counter. 15 seconds should heat the tea. (stands and waits for the bell to ring) Why is the bell ringing? Is someone at the door? No, no that is the microwave. Ah yes, warm tea. (Sits and drinks tea while looking around). I wonder why the mixer is on the counter. Mark doesn't clean up anything around here. (eyes fall on the note on the table—make cake) Ah yes, I had better make that cake or Mark will think I do nothing all day. (snips open the

package with the scissors on the counter and dumps it into the bowl).
Yes, I need milk, eggs, and oil. (walks to the fridge) What am I getting?
(Rereads the recipe) Milk. okay milk. How much? 1 1/4 cups. Where are
those measuring cups? (Slide, shut; slide, shut; slide shut, he opens and
closes the drawers and he sighs). Here they are. One cup. (slosh) 1/4 cup
(slosh) Did I put in the 1/4 cup or just one cup. (Re-measures the 1/4
cup). What am I doing? I usually put milk in my tea? What is this for?
Oh, yes, a cake—I'm making a cake. (Picks up the box with the recipe)
Oil? Where is that oil?

Just thinking about the process makes my head spin. Each
step is excruciating and painful when you cannot find things, or
remember whether or not you have completed a particular step in
the recipe. Three eggs could be placed in and mixed; and then in a
jumbled mess of memory lapse more eggs are plopped in and stirred.
Confusion, frustration, and stress accompany a once simple task.

Cooking is not many men's forte, or even in their skill set,
but my father could cook and BBQ whenever needed. Six months
preceding my mother's death from cancer, he cooked many of the
meals and would deliver them on a tray up to her. After his second
wife died, he picked up the chef's hat again very successfully. He
braised lake trout, fried chicken, and roasted beef cuts.

Not only are there losses in the basics of cooking and simple
tasks, but the very core of eating is disrupted in Alzheimer patients.
In the brain there is a sensor which is triggered by a message from
your stomach demanding food. The cable line announcing hunger
awareness is sent into crazy confusion during this disease takeover.

"I just ate. I'm not hungry," he would argue after my morning
visits which I usually ended by preparing his lunch. Other times,
after I successfully talk him into eating and finish cleaning up,
and then he would say, "I think it is time to eat." Arguing is often
not worth the trouble so the toaster gets a lot of use. Patience is a
necessary virtue to practice for caregiving.

When the process of cooking and the desire of eating has been tampered with, the concern of making sure your loved one has proper nutrition becomes paramount. To make matters worse the sensation of tasting is diminished, and swallowing becomes a difficult chore. Adding to this concern is the knowledge that choking is a very viable cause of death, but for today I think on the scripture which says, "Man shall not live by bread alone but by every word that proceeds from the mouth of God."[5]

The importance of daily food is necessary for physical well-being, but Jesus emphasizes the greater need to spiritually feast on the Word of God. My prayer is that as Dad goes down this journey of slowing food consumption, along with physical and mental deterioration, that somewhere in the reaches of his brain the stored scripture food which he has 'fed' on throughout his life will be the very spiritual food he needs to feed his soul through the difficult days ahead for him, and for me.

---

[5]   Matthew 4:4 King James Version

Chapter 8

LADIES AND LEMONS

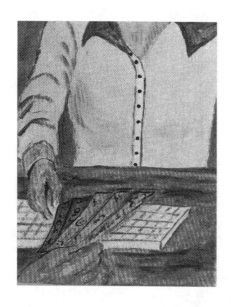

DAVID, MY ELDEST SIBLING, IS IN TOWN AND I NEED HIS HELP. WE stand at the door of a previous middle-aged bank teller's house. She had been Dad's favourite clerk though he always joked with all the bank ladies. He was always able to make conversation with anyone, but something of this situation smelled like day-old skunk roadkill. The remains are not there but the smell lingers. His willingness to lend a hand or give a handout was being baited. The worm dangling from the fishing line was friendship. Crossing the line between professional courtesy blurs when Dad begins to slip the bank lady money for her grown children and spend time with her strictly as a friend.

When going to the bank becomes as common as eating one's breakfast, I know I need to investigate his finances to assess where he stands. While I am discovering that big chunks of money have been withdrawn and he has no knowledge or remembrance of it, as well as no new purchases to show for it, the bank teller is being dismissed discreetly. His bank account resembles a closet in disarray and shoes are missing. We do not know how much has been swindled, but after some detective work, I discover he has also loaned this woman a large sum of money. With a bounced cheque in hand, we stand knocking at her door. She sounds so innocent and sincere that it almost fools me, but I hold my ground while David verbally pushes to make arrangement for repayment.

Anyone can take advantage of a gracious, kind person slipping into dementia because the person honestly doesn't remember, and if you play your cards right, you can hit the jack pot unless that is. . . there is a family member watching out for them. Few people are big time thieves at heart, but every clerk or cashier faces temptation when my dad arrives at the checkout. He pays and asks if he has paid and then insists while they are bagging the items that he hasn't paid while holding up another crisp twenty-dollar bill in his shaking hand.

Almost everything I learned about money, I learned from Father. How to make it, save it, and share it. I remember peering from behind my mother's robin-egg blue, A-line dress, eyes popping while Dad plopped down each week's pay.

"Barbie," he stated plainly— "this is for God." My mother dutifully handed the church envelope to him. After stuffing in some bills, she recorded the amount. "I think we need to give a little extra to . . ." and he named off a struggling missionary home on furlough or someone in need. "This is for savings, the mortgage, and groceries," he continued while scooping out the varied amounts for her to organize, record and balance. Most of the time there were few or no bills left on the table, unless he had sold an Electrolux recently, which led to him excitedly running his fingers through his hair and he would offer her to use the extra money wherever she saw fit. My mom, who appreciated how hard he worked for each dollar and his provision for all of us, organized the books with wisdom. If there was extra and the midnight madness sales were on at the Hudson Bay Company, I giggled and grinned knowing I'd get to stay up late and fight the crowds with Mom and may even be able to wear a new dress on Sunday to church.

Some Saturday afternoons in the summer, I went with my father to Trail's End, a local market selling fresh produce. I held his hand while my runners would slap the dirt on the path. As a city girl, this was so different for me than shopping with my mom in the supermarket. Chickens squawked in the background and globs of blood red meat lay behind clouded curved glass counters while stall owners shouted out their bargain prices.

It was near closing time and an older man with a dried apple-prune face hollered, "One dollar for the box". Lemons remind me of freshly cleaned rooms or lemon dust spray on polished dark wood dressers.

Before I knew what was happening, my father stepped forward, "I'll take them all off your hands, ten dollars for all the boxes of lemons you have left."

I counted using my peter pointer —fifteen boxes. I'm sure my father had already sized up his haul.

"Sure," the man said, and my father handed me one of the many boxes.

"Now the car is right outside those doors. Watch out for leaving cars, and I'll be right behind you," he beamed as though he had just won the lottery even though he wasn't a gambler.

He carried some boxes. After two more trips each, we jumped into the car which had never smelled that clean and fresh before.

"What are we going to do with all of these lemons?" I queried.

"Sell them," he stated matter of fact. I smiled at the prospect of business. My Kool aid stand hadn't done well the Saturday before, but I knew if my father said we would sell all the lemons—we would. I would be his salesgirl. I gleefully grinned in anticipation as we drove home. Most of our neighbours probably would never buy lemons again all summer, I thought at the end of the evening while stacking the empty boxes.

During the early younger years, parents wisely spend their income to raise a family and save what they can. Now they desperately need those grown children to help them wisely care for that money —ever watching for people who might take advantage of them.

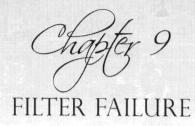

FILTER FAILURE

THE FIRST TIME I WENT TO A TALK REGARDING ALZHEIMER'S, I came out a blubbering mess. The speaker spewed out rude comments to shock the audience of caregivers.

"So how will you respond when your parent or spouse swears a 'blue streak' or yells in loud outbursts in the mall about the size of some woman's bosom using words that young men might snicker about in locker rooms?" the well-dressed speaker asks while clicking to the next power point slide.

My face falls. To paraphrase one of the bullet points of her 'talk', she communicated how the diseased mind is no longer eighty years plus but reverts to a twenty-year-old with the filter part of the mind removed. Their raw, naked thoughts will streak across their mind and may come out streaming in an R-rated fashion. At this point of the journey my dad is not there, and I pray that his Christianity will be so deep in his soul that I won't have to face that. Yet I realize that such a time may come.

I remember my nana who had become a Christian late in life through the witness of my mother. She traversed this stage in her dementia in wild flashes of horrid colour. Her words normally were filled with grace and as her granddaughter, I had spent many weeks of my summer vacation in Toronto with her as I was growing up. These times were filled with trips to the Toronto Zoo, Casa Loma, baking cookies and craft filled afternoons. She was a doting grandmother. However, the demonic claws of dementia tore at the core of who she was, as she morphed into a crazed old woman in her later years.

My parents had to cope with this disease many years before my father ever developed it. One day we checked on Nana, who insisted that she could still live alone having moved to London. Standing in my grandmother's living room, my mother's face drenched with tears, she whispered to my father, "Get Carolyn out of here. Don't let her see." But it was too late for that; I had come in the back door. Sagging bulges of flesh flapped on my nana's boney frame as she streaked by swearing, "I'll never go into a @#$%^ home and why the @#$%@ didn't you come when I called!?"

The withered old woman looked haggish, pathetic, and scary; this was a shell that once housed a wonderful lady. I cannot dread the thought that Mr. Hyde will invade my father, so I force myself to enjoy the Dr. Jekyll for the present. The filter is mostly holding, but every now and then a small barrage of inappropriate comments slips through revealing Mr. Hyde's presence.

My father loves children and always has. He bussed kids to church, collecting runny- nosed forgotten children from neglected neighbourhoods, and lifting them onto the Sunday School bus where he took them to hear about Jesus. I am sure some children received more attention and love in those half hour rides to and from church than in their whole weekend. Kids loved my father and climbed all over him like monkeys on trees. They told him about their pets, their friends, and troubles at home. He often brought snacks when he began to realize that many of them were coming without having eaten breakfast.

He still smiles whenever he sees little children. Recently my dad notices a dark haired little girl standing by her mom when he innocently says, "You're so cute I could take you home with me." The tiny girl smiles shyly but begins to back up behind her mother's patterned leggings. The mother glares at me and turns while visually throwing darts at the 'supposed' dirty old man. Maybe in her past some older man had abused her, or maybe because our world is so tainted with the fear of pedophiles, she misjudged the elderly man's innocent but poorly worded comment.

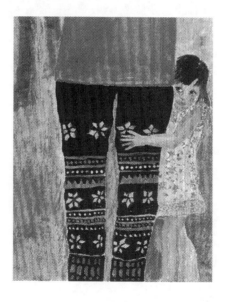

Attempting to undo the awkward moment, I quickly interject, "He just thinks she is a cute little girl." At that moment I was humbled, embarrassed, and hurt for him. He stands oblivious to the entire interchange. Later I try to explain how he needs to be careful about what he says. He staunchly defends his innocence, looks disgusted and then hurt that I or the woman would think such a thing. I do not think poorly of him. I know his heart.

— ❋ —

"I know what abuse is," he murmurs. Here I am a grown woman listening to my dad recollect a story I do not think he had ever pulled out of his memory closet to share before. "When I was fifteen, I came to Ontario from Nova Scotia to be a farm hand for the summer," he begins. "That summer I baled hay and shovelled mountains of manure from dawn to dusk. There was a man about forty, an old farmhand I guess," his face began to change, and he looks through me as if he is being transported to that night which he is about to tell me. "The man, who rarely said anything to us young boys, creaked open my bedroom door and headed towards my bed. He tried to get in bed with me, but that wasn't going to be happening to me!" His face is fierce, and I sit, a little shell shocked, as he continues. "The next day, I told the farmer about what the old farmhand tried to do, and I never saw him after that." Transporting back into the present he looks me in the eye and says, "Don't you ever let anyone try to touch one of those kids of yours." Stunned and embarrassed I try to process the revelation. It was an odd conversation to have with one's Dad. However, I know that his high respect for women and children defines him. Even if one day the verbal filter fails, and he says things that he shouldn't, I know who he is and trust his heart.

Chapter 10

VACUUMS AND MAGGOTS

When most wives empty out their husband's pants pockets before laundry day, pens, Kleenex, and maybe keys are retrieved, but my mother regularly removed filthy six-inch square cloths which were pristine white before being used as a vacuum cleaner demonstration. The black round spot of medieval chimney-looking soot covering each cloth was popped into the washing machine. Just as my father worked two jobs most of his life, (driving a city bus full time and selling Electrolux part time), he had two purposes when working. He loved the thrill of closing a deal when selling vacuums to provide for his family and the joy of sharing his love for Jesus Christ with as many people on the bus or in their homes. He not only showed them how they could have a clean house, but more importantly, he showed them how they could stand before a holy God with a clean heart.

Today, a door-to-door salesman is viewed as obnoxious, almost unprofessional, but in the sixties, seventies and early eighties it was definitely a wise way to do business. I remember my father encouraging me to sell Fuller Brush products when I was in high school. I enjoyed meeting various elderly couples and stay-at-home moms. I never quite inherited his salesmanship though.

Father would often spend Saturday mornings out selling when

both adults would most likely be home. Although my father could sell water to a fish, he felt it was important to only make the sale if the person truly needed it and could afford his Electrolux machine. He would often allow them to trade in their old vacuums to reduce their cost. All the while he would calculate the cost of replacement parts and the resale value of their old model. On one particular Saturday he could taste success, but the price was a bit out of reach for the couple.

"I'll tell you what I'll do," he said, looking discreetly around. "I can knock off more money if you have something else you want me to take for trade."

One might think by the way he talked that he was an explorer trading in the New World, and at that very moment my father's eyes landed on the gun over the fireplace.

"How long has it been since you went hunting?" my dad directed the question to the man of the house.

It seemed a random question, maybe even a tactic to distract, but the lady of the house understood, and she quickly answered for her husband.

"He hasn't shot anything in years," she pitched in before he even had a chance to catch onto the trade deal that was unfolding around him.

"Well, she's right," he concurred, his eyes lingering over the piece. The lights flickered in his mind too, and he shot out the idea as though it was his own original thought. "How much would you take off the vacuum for the gun?" he queried as he reached and pulled the gun down from over the mantle. They closed the deal.

As I helped him unpack his wares that afternoon and the sun's rays glinted off the stock of his 'new gun', it was easy to see from the opened back gate of the station wagon what he had acquired.

— ❋ —

My mind shoots into the present as I drive up the driveway and see the rear hatch of his Jeep up. It was not the station wagon, but he was leaning into the back of the vehicle just like he had done so many years ago after a morning of sales. With that memory fresh in my mind, I jump out of my mini van, pondering the day's activities which I had planned for us this morning. I walk toward the opened hatch when my eyes widen. I was about to ask what treasure he had in the back of his truck when I see. . .. The rear 'whitish' carpet appears to be vibrating —no it is alive with creamy white——AHHHH!

Like a squirrel on the road about to be mowed down, I stop and gasp, "Maggots? Why? How? Disgusting!" The milky white mass mull about like shoppers in a crowded mall at Christmas. "What happened?" I stammer.

"I don't know. I was trying to find keys to drive to your place, but Mark must have taken them," he replies.

After he lost his licence three weeks ago, my brother and I thought that we had completely locked up the vehicle, but the back-hatch door must not have been completely shut because Dad had slipped a garbage bag in the back of the vehicle thinking he would drive it to the dump later. Later never came.

"I don't know where they've come from," he continues.

Looking around in the backyard, I spot the black garbage bag covered with hundreds of clinging maggots which he must have removed from the vehicle but forgotten moments before I drove up. He could not remember ever having put a garbage bag in the back of the jeep weeks earlier or even having removed the bag that morning only minutes before I arrived. He loves things to be clean and I desperately try not to throw up. The original day's plan which was to stop at the thrift store before a walk in the park to feed the ducks is now exchanged for scooping, whisking, and finally vacuuming maggots.

While cleaning them up I think about my bug collection on my living room walls. I love the beauty of nature, but these are revolting creatures that seem to be without beauty and purpose, yet I know in my scientific mind this isn't true. Maggots eat dead flesh and can be used to heal physical wounds by cleaning out the dead infected tissue. As we roll the maggots with our gloved hands into a mound, these brain shaped blobs nauseate me. I imagine maggots eating the dying memories in my dad's brain leaving less and less of him. There is no cure, no way back here on earth. He is dying slowly, and the mind is being eaten, but there is a hope, an eternal hope since he knows the ultimate cleaner. Just like the washing machine cleaned dirt from the sample cloth, Jesus Christ washed away my dad's sin through faith. Jesus' resurrection is the truth that secures a home in heaven for him to be raised and live forever with a new mind, heart, and body totally restored.

Chapter 11

WANDERING AND HOME

'You are here'. Every shopping mall map posts this obvious statement. If every road were straight with exactly the same-coloured houses lining the streets, then you would never be able to find your way through a city. Geography is about the variation of landforms, rock outcroppings, fish shaped ponds, or a stand of pine trees. To navigate around the world, you must be acutely aware of your surroundings. "Ah yes, on this corner there is a Tim Horton's Donut Shop, a gas station, and that big oak tree that looks like a gnarled number seven reaching up into the clouds." Through recognition of landmarks, you know where you are. Once you have established that very important fact, quite often you know which streets you need to travel home, which corners to turn left on, or which short cut to take through a park. Repeated trips in the past will help you find home quickly. My dad's home is the welcoming red brick back-split with a glass, floral-patterned door. My dad would never have picked that door, but his deceased wife liked it; this is home.

Imagine you stare at what used to be a familiar corner, but now you feel like you have been parachuted out of a plane and dropped into another city or Mars, for all you know. You have no memories of this store or gas station where you regularly used to get gas. You are in a fog. A fog in the early morning of a crisp fall day is mysterious and haunting, but the morning ball of fire will streak through the mist dissipating it like an empty room after the crowd has left. Yet, for my dad and others who stagger in the fog of dementia, it rarely lifts. It isn't burnt off. It thickens like a smothering blanket. His inner GPS and locator are offline. *Where am I? How do I get home?* These are questions which lead to panic seizing any shimmering memories that might flicker hope.

I lost two men, in one weekend. After all I am the sandwiched generation. My teen boys are not extremely extroverted, but they are friendly and used to their mom's wild and creative ideas to make memories and money. I love being a stay-at-home mom who homeschooled her children. Now, maybe, it is time to head back into the work force, yet I have an aging father who needs care and I know that teens only pretend they don't need you around. Since I love young people and feel it would be a great opportunity for my family to learn about other cultures, I talk my husband and three sons into plunging into an adventure together. We would be a homestay for a teen boy coming from Brazil to learn English.

Our Sunday morning routine is running on schedule when the phone chirps through the noisy buzz.

"Hello," I answer not really listening. My eyes grow wide as I scoot to a quieter room to understand what the man is telling me.

"There's a boy here with a paper with your name and number on it," the officer states.

"We'll be right there! Wait! Where is he? We were supposed to be picking up a boy on Tuesday at the airport," my words rush together.

My husband and I jump into the red truck and whisk through the streets of London while I explain that this was our new student who had arrived two days early and was wandering the streets of our midsized south-western Ontario city looking for us. As we drive up, the hooded eighteen-year-old is awkwardly standing beside a large suitcase, holding an overstuffed backpack, and gripping a crumpled paper with his new home location. He must have walked a few kilometres before realizing he was helpless and lost and at the mercy of everyone and anyone. Shaken but with a brave face pasted on, he half smiles at us, thankful to be found. I had seen that same face on my dad earlier that weekend.

Whether eighteen and lost in a foreign city where you do not speak the language, or eighty-one and lost in your own neighbourhood of many years, lost is scary and found is wonderful.

"I will get out here," my dad firmly says with determination just before I turn the car to take him down his street. "You took me all the way to the cottage, and I know you need to get home to your family. I can walk down the street so you can keep going home."

"Are you sure?" I ask, knowing that stubborn voice. I knew it is a bad decision, but I give in to a moment of my selfishness and pull into the Home Hardware store parking lot. All he must do is cross the busy main street and walk straight down a block and a half, fifteen houses at best, I rationalize. People with dementia wander, but those are the ones who are in locked units. My dad is not ready to be a mouse in a labyrinth. He has never been lost before, but he is usually with me or my brother. I pull into the familiar hardware store parking lot, and he gets out waving me on. He will be fine; I shushed my inner second guesser.

Steam puffs out from under the pot lids of the rushed dinner I am preparing when the phone rings. Mark usually calls around dinner to ask how the day went with dad as he takes over the 'evening shift'. He lives there and Dad appreciates his presence, and I am glad too, or we would have had to seek different arrangements.

"Hello," the phone presses against my cheek as I lift the lid to stir the contents of dinner.

"No, I dropped him off an hour ago. What do you mean he's not home?" Like Jell-O left on the counter my thoughts and emotions spread in every direction. Guilt and worry overtake. It was a crisp late October evening and he had been wandering for over an hour. Ghoulish fingers of dread squeeze my heart within my chest. He must feel like he is in a corn maze of houses not knowing which way to go. I hang up the phone, turn off the stove, and grab the keys.

I drive back over, looking down every street between his house and mine. Most of us have looked for a missing pet, but this was a man, Dad, the man who knew every intersection in the city because he had waited along the roads, drove competently around and through the streets for years on his bus. This man was lost!

"Where should I go next?" I burst through the back door begging to be directed.

My brother's relief shone through, "He's home."

I repeated my brother's words with a sigh. I listened as Mark explain how someone from our church saw him pushing a bicycle down Second street about a mile and half from home in the wrong direction.

Dad interrupts the story, "I am fine. I found a nice old bike on the side of the road which someone was throwing out and I decided to bring it home."

Then he stared into his cupful of tea while Mark ran downstairs to get something. In my brother's absence Dad confided, "Carolyn, I admit, I don't know what happened. I honestly did not know where I was and you know . . ." he stopped mentally searching for the name of the man who had driven him home, "you know the man from our church who works at the grocery store, he drove me home."

"Dale Neff," I say, filling in the blank, not wanting to tax his already flustered brain. He was home but this would only be the beginning of his wanderings.

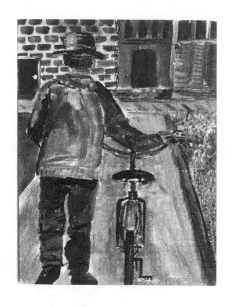

Chapter 12

HONKING HORNS

RUSHING; I INHERITED THIS TRAIT FROM MY FATHER, IF YOU COULD call it a trait. There is a thrill in trying to accomplish ten things when there is only time for five. After crushing my right pointer finger with a sledgehammer, I discovered I had another hand and was forced to use it. What a blessing in disguise, because now I am ambidextrous when doing the laundry or serving the dinner. I am constantly challenging myself to increase the number of activities I can complete simultaneously.

My father loved the adrenaline of the 'rush' or he acted as though he did because that is how 'the MacBains' operated. Every morning he needed to be at the bus station at 5:15 am. The alarm would ring at five. The house became a stadium of lights.

"Where is my belt? I thought my shirt was on the bedpost. Have you got the lunch ready, Barbie?" the barrage of questions fired from the upstairs bedroom across the hall from mine. Heavy feet thumped down the carpeted stairs. Dishes clattered while the lunch pail was pulled out of the cupboard. The steamy kettle whistled calling for attention. Clang! The thermos tipped. This daily repeated routine of 'rush' intensified if he had slept in, even a few minutes. The noise factor doubled, usually waking me up but not my brothers because they could sleep through a tornado pitching cow bells through the house. I would often slip down the stairs to watch the flurry of activity and sometimes was part of the assembly line handing him his bus jacket or cap as he flew out the door into the car. If my mother wasn't in the car ready to give him a ride, he tapped the horn. I'm sure our neighbours disposed of their alarm clocks because our house became a beacon of noise and light at such a horribly early time.

Most people rarely use a horn in a vehicle except for real emergencies. Horn blowing had many purposes though for my father. When our family purchased a new-to-us family car, father used the horn more often in the beginning so we would be able to distinguish its particular sound. If a family member was being picked up from piano lessons, the library, or youth group, two short taps of the horn was your cue to come running. One might think that the family quirk was confined to family life, but no.

My father's bus horn, a much throatier sounding beep, was as important as the air brakes on the bus. His favourite bragging rite is probably because of his well used horn, "I've never had an at fault accident in 40 years and one week."

Honking was not just for avoiding accidents or waving to another passing driver, he often used it for his passengers as well. If he realized that one of his patrons was not at their regular stop, maybe because they were running late, which he seemed to totally identify with, then his horn was there for the rescue. He often knew where regular passengers lived or the corner they would be coming from, and he would roll ahead to that location and give a loud blast. People responded just like us kids. They flew out from behind their door and sprinted for their ride.

"Good morning, I see you're running a bit behind. Do not worry, it is a brand-new day. His mercies are new every morning."

They probably wondered whose mercies he was referring to. They would soon learn if they travelled daily with him because he was never shy about his God. They panted and smiled, thankful to have not missed the bus, all because of that horn. Many mornings he drove singing an off-tune rendition of the chorus "Heavenly Sunshine" especially if the morning sun was streaming in across his windshield. During my years of catching the bus to the local university (of which Dad made sure he was the driver) I remember thinking how embarrassing his singing was. Yet looking back through the gates of time, I realize that it brought a smile to the lives of harried people. Everyone loved that cheerful driver!

My father could strip off roof shingles in record time, rebuild a vacuum cleaner in a few hours, and find the most efficient way to drive across the city in under thirty minutes. However, age has a way of catching up with our busyness and slowing us down. Speed and time were synonymous. Now his walking is deliberate, his thinking is slowed, and I am glad he is not driving any more because his response time would be as molasses on a cold day. Horn blowing was his trait, his trademark, but during his last few months of driving, horns were blowing at him when he misjudged the distance between his car and the car in the adjacent lane. HONK! HONK!

Sometimes when he walks across his once quiet suburban street in a snail-like fashion, he is oblivious to the increased traffic on the way from the Tim Horton's on the corner. If their horns could yell, they would scream, "Get off the road, old man!" BEEP, swerve HONK! Drivers are crass and maybe even rude, but the reality is, he probably does need to get off the road in more ways than one.

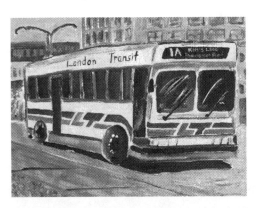

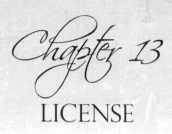

LICENSE

SIXTEEN, A MAGICAL NUMBER! I TWIRLED AROUND LIKE A BALLERINA in a pink tutu squealing while wearing plain jeans, mud brown top, and dirty runners, "I passed! I got it!"

A driver's license is one of the first rites of passage to adulthood-independence! Just months before my 16th birthday, on a holiday at my aunt's farm, I was behind the wheel of my grandpa's old lemon-yellow Buick gripping the steering wheel with leech-like fingers. I maneuvered slowly down the bumpy gravel quarter-mile laneway under my father's directions.

"Look at the hood ornament and it should line up with the right side of the edge of the driveway and that will get you started, but then you must look ahead to where you are going." My father had trained multiple people how to drive a bus and I was just another trainee, his daughter in a big car. The yellow lines, the mirrors, the shoulder checks were all part of my driving lesson with Father. My mother had the heavy foot with aggressive driving skills which I inherited, but my father had the patience to teach and the nerve to sit in the passenger seat while I learned to merge into traffic, check for blind spots and parallel park. I never did learn to parallel park well because who ever heard of a city bus being parallel parked.

— ❀ —

"I drove a city bus for forty years and one week and never had an at-fault accident," my dad brags to the doctor. Many bus drivers weren't as attentive or were careless, but not my father. Whether on ice, in fog, or traversing through a snowstorm he had managed to make his bus go and stop exactly where he wanted it to. Driving a city bus in a sea of cars is like maneuvering an oil tanker through a narrow canal filled with canoes. For 40 years Father successfully kept control of his bus and was awarded for his many years of perfect driving.

"Mr. MacBain," the doctor declares without emotion, "I had to contact the Ontario Ministry of Driving regarding your test score on the cognitive test that you took a few weeks ago. You no longer can drive. Do you remember taking that test?"

"Well," silence filled the air, "yes," he slowly affirms, his brow furrows as he tries to recollect the contents of the test.

You didn't score so well on the test. It is a memory test and a cognitive judgment test," the doctor pushes on.

"Well, old people like me forget some things, but what does that have to do with driving?" Frustration and understanding begin to rise. "You can't tell a man who's driven a bus all his life without an accident that he can't drive his car because he can't remember a few things. That's just not right!" his voice intensifies.

Holding his hand up the doctor repeats firmly but patiently, "I administered the test. It shows that your memory is poor and since this condition might affect your driving . . ."

"What test?" Dad mutters interrupting the doctor's coming explanation.

"Don't you remember taking the test, Dad?" I interrogate cautiously, looking from my dad to the doctor.

Avoiding my question, Dad directs his question to the doctor while trying to gain control, "So what does this mean? I just need to be careful when I drive. My license is not gone. You are just concerned, right?" The look in his eyes was one of confusion, anger, and fear, much like a kid in a principal's office who is not sure why he is there. It was as though the past conversation had not taken place and the doctor begins again to re-explain the test he had given, the failed result, and the removal of the license. Each point is challenged, argued, and then forgotten within moments. With patience expended, the doctor ends the conversation when he realizes it would do no good to talk through the merry-go-round again.

Head spinning, we leave. The ride in the elevator fills me with questions which I leave hanging in the air because to answer them would be like popping endless balloons. Would he really understand that his license was taken? Would he accept it? Would he remember? For the first week I keep him busier than usual. My brother did his part by hiding his car keys and removing the battery out of the car. Week two, however, was not so easy. Every morning the conversation on the phone would roughly follow the same pattern. He would ask what we were doing that day and would suggest driving over.

"No, Dad you can't drive. The doctor took your license. I'll come over and get you and we can . . ." I cannot finish my plan of distraction before he interrupts.

"I have my license! It's right here in my wallet. What do you mean I cannot drive? Mark and you must be up to something." Despite my best efforts his response is always the same.

I try not to take the bait but would inevitably get caught in a cycle of explaining, arguing, and explaining again, which would end in angry frustration leading to an 80-year-old's tantrum often expressed in a rush of words.

"I'm going to the license bureau to find out what's going on! It's my car!! I want my keys and I'm going to drive!!!" With that ultimatum the dial tone would buzz over the line. Quickly, I scoop up my keys to drive over knowing that I will find him in his car trying all the keys in the ignition to find the right one. After coaxing him out of the driver's seat of his car and into the passenger seat of mine, we head out. Arriving at my home, we garden, cut trees, or chisel off bricks for landscaping. The morning goes by repeating stories and chatting about his childhood. Some stories I do not ever recall hearing as he pulls ancient treasures out. I take joy in the moments of work and story telling knowing that tomorrow I will face the driving argument again. For the present, I enjoy the moment.

Losing the privilege to drive is like clipping a bird's wings. Many elderly people lose their driver's license, and it takes time to accept and adjust to the loss and the new limitations. However, for the dementia patient the loss must be relived, adjusted to every single day, because each day they learn the news for the <u>first</u> time.

Chapter 14

JUGGLING NOT DROWNING

CARE GIVING IS DIFFERENT THAN VOLUNTARILY ENJOYING AN afternoon together working, building, or walking around a garden centre. I often find myself doing these same activities with my father, but it is different when you *are* his social life and you *must* plan activities to keep him busy every day. I remember, as a twelve-year-old girl, when my father spent a few hours with me one evening teaching me to juggle, first using oranges and tangerines, and then moving to hard-boiled eggs. Juggling three objects is hard because there must always be one up in the air. It can be done, but it requires practiced skill. For two years, my brother and I have been juggling caregiving non-stop. Mark comes home from work, and he resides in my dad's home. Mark makes the meal, and they eat supper together, watch TV, or just pass the time together. As things began to progress, I needed to invite my dad over almost once a day to break up his day, and after he lost his license, I would go over and visit or drive him some place to give him something to do daily.

Juggling involves three balls. As a married woman with children, I juggle keeping a household running. The second ball is outside my home involving loving and serving extended family and friends inside and outside of the church. The third major ball is me. I need to do things just for me: Bible devotions, physical exercise, and hobbies. The real difficulty comes when a person you are caring for is part of every ball in the juggling routine. In the beginning as my dad needed me to become his social activity calendar, I try to include him in my regular daily world.

"Do you want to help me chop a young sapling from behind the rose of Sharon?" He always enjoys such mornings, but it becomes increasingly hard to dream of projects without dropping one of the balls.

It is necessary for a caregiver to recognize when <u>too much</u> has become overwhelming. A plan for a break away is necessary or all the balls will drop to the floor rolling in every direction.

"Hello, are you open to an idea?" I ask in desperation talking to my girlfriend on the phone. "I know you are looking at building a business of cleaning houses, and I know you know my dad. Would you want to come and work two afternoons a week? Technically you can do some cleaning but feel free to make him tea and just pass some of the time with him chatting."

For each caregiver, this process of getting a respite and have some rest is necessary. It will look different for each family due to the snail pace with which this disease progresses. Help is needed for the long haul of loving, caring, and making it to the end whole and without regrets on all fronts.

Childhood vacations were fun-filled. On one vacation fun almost ended in disaster. My eldest brother was off at his own camp, but the rest of the family headed out for our camping trip. My mother never enjoyed true camping in a tent or trailer, but she could handle a cabin. The little blue painted clapboard cabin would make a perfect home for a week. We hiked and fished in the nearby creek. It was a wonderful week until Thursday. My father, being adventurous, decided to take my brother and me to a special place.

I was squealing with delight standing in my yellow bathing suit and Mark, four years my senior, had a red towel draped around his neck ready to go too.

"You be careful with those kids," warned my mother. "It is rough waters."

Jumping out of the car, I gawked. I had seen bubbling, rocky rivers on the Wonderful World of Disney TV series which aired Sunday evenings at 6 pm. We always got to watch 45 minutes of the hour program, before we had to leave for evening Church at 7 pm. I often created my own ending for each story, making up some wild ones. Now here in front of me was a river like the one in the story about a bear who came to drink in the cool eddies and ended up making friends with a boy. I imagined I was in a Disney set.

"What are we going to do? It's too rough to swim." I half announced, half asked.

At the very moment, a dad and a boy came careening from behind some rocks laughing while being carried along. Extreme fun and terror melded together in my mind.

Incredulously Mark exclaimed, "We are going to do THAT?" pointing toward the rushing current of teens coming next.

We watched as each group of kids, family, or teens rode the current down the middle and splashed into the ending eddy where the ride's slight natural slope levelled.

"Now hold on to me and don't let go," Dad commanded.

There was no need to state the obvious. Mark's eyes, round as pancakes, reflected fear and excitement. We climbed to the top where everyone was getting in, and I clung to my father like a baby koala to its mother. My brother did the same. Fear gripped me like shrink wrap on packages when we entered the stream. My brother's and my grip tightened around our father's throat as the water splashes attacked us. Where was my father's head? In our desperation to hold tight, he was forced below the water only bobbing occasionally for air. He realized his own children would drown him if he did not do something. That something was severe, shocking, and frightening. He pushed with all his might and shoved us away. Our screaming was unheard because the roaring water swallowed the sound. But my father emerged like a hippo surviving a crocodile attack. Using strong arms, he scooped us back into himself, but this time we were facing outward. He was our lifesaver at that moment.

As I reflect, I realize that he needed to save himself or we all would have been in trouble. Care giving can have a drowning effect and casting them away for a short time to avoid drowning is often necessary to keep the balls aloft and to survive.

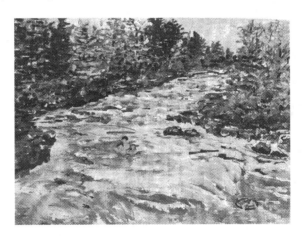

Chapter 15

PETS AND OUR HUMANITY

CATS PURR CONTENTEDLY, DOGS WAG TAILS EXCITEDLY, BIRDS SING sweetly, even fish swish blithely. The word pet is a noun, but it can also be a verb meaning to caress and stroke. Not everyone has a Lassie dog which follows the boy everywhere he goes and licks his face, a young lad's dream companion, but my father was one of the lucky ones who had such a dog named Teddy.

Growing up in Nova Scotia on a farm and being the youngest of many, father needed that special someone. Brothers were just brothers. Once they decided that it was time their little brother learned to swim, and they pushed him into a swirling river, and he had to learn quickly before he was dragged down stream toward the mill! While his brothers and sisters were extremely bright and talented, he always struggled to read and write. But Teddy understood and Teddy didn't care. This young boy often visited his favourite fishing hole after school with Teddy trotting alongside. The loyal dog accompanied him almost everywhere. One time, however, when the boy (my father) was out in the back forty without his dog and he came to the fast-flowing water, he looked across and there was his dog tracking him. Teddy saw him and leaped into the water swimming with his head bobbing like a moving log going down stream. The boy ran alongside the bank while the swimming, swirling dog was dragged down stream. When the tired dog finally dragged himself up on the shore, he shook himself wildly and then jumped up onto him and they both flopped on the ground relieved and happy. Drenched and exhausted the two walked side by side all the way home. Like Mary and her little lamb, everywhere that the boy went, the dog was sure to follow. Teddy truly was a storybook pet. There was no cleaning up after his messes. As a farm dog, he'd run out to the back field to fertilize the farmland, and best of all, he slept at the bottom of his bed keeping the young boy's feet warm during those long Maritime winter nights.

I could see in my dad's eyes the longing for a pet when my cat came to the door, dog-like, waiting to be petted. Dad would find a comfortable chair in my house and stroke the fluffy old thing.

Owning a dog or cat in the city is more complex and things do not always go so smoothly. My family loves our white long-haired cat. One day, however, he simply decided he didn't want to regularly use the kitty litter. Finding a random pile of stinky clothes on the floor ready for the laundry or a soft bunched up blanket on a bed, our cat left us smelly, gooey treasures throughout the house. After trying everything we could think of and every suggestion from Google, we decided the cat needed to go. After asking Dad for advice, he agreed that maybe it would be best. One Friday evening before we were going to have the cat done away with, I decided to try one last crazy idea. Why not make the kitty litter box much bigger by using a huge rubber tote with no lid? The problem was resolved. I love that big fat cat and so does my dad.

"I am glad you figured it out," I heard him whisper sympathetically as he scratched the ears of the pet who almost wasn't.

Dad, too, is struggling with the basics of toiletry. In dementia the part of the brain that signals you to get moving toward the great white throne stops working intermittently. There is no warning, no sensation. It is totally unfair and rather embarrassing. I know there have been times when I am going over to take him out for the morning, and he is up in the washroom for a very long time.

"I'll be down in a few minutes," he mumbles.

I can guess what had happened because I see a pile of clumped-up sheets thrown to the bottom of the stairs and a few days before I saw freshly washed under garments hanging on the shower curtain rod. Quietly, I wait in the kitchen and feel his shame. He comes down the stairs not wanting to give an explanation to his daughter for his tardiness. He simply looks down. The same look he and the cat had shared. I wish he had an animal at his house to pet, to stroke, to confide in about the unfairness of getting old.

I considered getting Dad a dog but walking him in the city every day and forgetting whether you had taken the dog for a walk, or not, might result in puddles on the floor or one exhausted old man and an over-walked dog. This does not even take into consideration the thought of them both getting lost. No, a cat might be better but after our difficulties with our cat, I settled on a fish. Fish cannot be petted, but they have the power to mesmerize and bring their own type of relaxation and comfort. Watching the creature scoot or float lazily across the glass with its tail fins spreading beautifully can bring moments of comfort and enjoyment.

I showed up at the door one day with Bob. It was an aquamarine blue Betta. I was excited.

"What would I want a fish for?" Dad asked incredulously.

"He's cute. His name is Bob. You will love him." I announced.

We spent the morning setting up the new fish in its dish with rocks and plants and a little light. After discussing Bob's food, we both plopped down in the two rose-coloured wing-backed chairs to watch Dad's new pet swim.

"Whenever I am not here, you can watch Bob."

Mark grew to love the little guy and talking to him became part of the routine for both my brother and Dad. However, Dad wasn't just talking to him when I wasn't in the room, he was feeding him. Anyone who knows about Betta fish understands that overfeeding can be a problem.

"I did not feed him!" Dad argues with Mark.

I stare in at the fish whose tummy had a growth resembling a tumour. His stomach dragged on the bottom and he seemed to struggle to swim to the top and then he struggled to swim to the bottom over the next few days. The constipated, overfed fish was not happy. After a few days it was all over. I immediately went out and purchased Bob the second, but this time we hid the food and his new companion is doing well. He swims beautifully and effortlessly bringing joy to Dad.

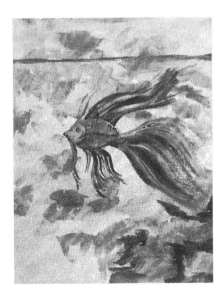

For an outing, I take Dad to the pet store with me. He thrills at all the creatures and even comments on the old leathery turtle for sale. He has been getting more tired and less able to walk around the aisles in the pet store; maybe he identifies with the old tortoise. I turn to browse the fish shelf for more supplies when I discover Dad is gone. I knew he was just talking to one of the patrons, but since I was engrossed in reading the directions on the blood worm treats for fish, I didn't notice that the conversation happening around me had ceased. Frantically I look around the store.

"Dad? Dad?"

No one answered.

"Were you the one just talking to the elderly gentleman just a moment ago?" I query several people in the store.

"Yes, I was just speaking to an older man," the last man responded. He steers me in the direction of where he thought my dad went. By this point the cashier and several shoppers were aiding me in the search when we all congregated together around the far corner of the store and see him.

He had sat down on a tall, now very compacted, pile of dog beds and had dozed off. Smiles spread across faces at the candid camera moment. The old man was about to topple over when the store owner reached out his hand to help him up to his feet.

God whispers his love to the lonely and calms the agitated soul with comforting words from his love letter. He instituted family to love and care for us, but he also created soft cuddly loving pets like cats and dogs and colourful fish to help bring a smile to our souls.

Chapter 16

LAUGH OR CRY

STRESS IS RUMOURED TO BE THE ROOT OF MANY AILMENTS, DISEASES, and disorders. Stress can accompany job loss, financial struggles, relationship issues, or care giving for a loved one. Stress is defined as crushing pressure which weighs on the mind affecting the body. Anyone who is honest about care giving for an Alzheimer's loved one must include the word stress. In the beginning of the journey, the family must figure out who can help, how they can help, when they can be available to care for the person with Alzheimer's to keep that person feeling loved and safe.

The stress continues and grief crowds in as you begin to lose the person you know. Seminars state that your loved one will be physically present but mentally unavailable. How can I or others endure such a long and draining parting? Sudden endings to life cause the grieving process to begin fully but extended sicknesses leading to death make the process of grieving a lengthier journey. I cry when another brain compartment collapses and the person I know is slowly being closed off. Somewhere inside, the real person is housed. I weep as he is being lost. As we lose, we wrestle to move forward into each new reduced future. I can choose to do it morbidly, dragging the family to death's checkered finish line, or we can celebrate family memories on the way. Though I know his blank stares may haunt me and other family members, we choose to still visit, and retell family memories. The celebration of life does not have to be encapsulated into a few five-minute eulogies at the funeral. Today we will sit on his bed and walk the children down memory lanes. It might even bring a moment of smile to his face, and it may bring laughter to the heavy hearts of his grandchildren and caregivers alike.

Most of our family's hilarious stories occurred on vacations. I was out with my mom on what proved to be one of the craziest summer afternoons on a camping vacation. My father was one of the three stooges, while my brothers would play their parts perfectly in what could be entitled a misadventure episode of laundering money. In the 1970's credit cards were used somewhat, but my father was a firm believer in cash. His wallet bulged like a jumbo submarine sandwich with lettuce-like American green cash and coloured Canadian money. The drive had been long. After setting up camp, Father was in definite need of an outhouse. Not wanting to spend any extra time in the smelly boxed building he quickly did his business and began to pull up his pants when plop! Oh no, he thought as he peered down the hole only to see his sandwich wallet of cash laying on top of the fresh deposit. Assessing the situation, he felt all was not lost because the waste sits in a holding tank about four feet down until there is a certain weight reached. Then the door will swing open, and the waste will drop into the main holding tank much deeper.

"Mark, come quick!" Father hollered, "Stand guard and do not let anyone use this outhouse. I have got to get a stick to reach my wallet. Our money for this whole trip is in there," he pointed toward the hole. He returned out of breath with tree branches in hand. "You can go. I got this." he announces confidently.

Mark was only too happy to be outside in the fresh air exploring the nearby forest behind the cabin. Meanwhile Father stuck his head down into the hole and with both knees on the wooden toilet seat, he managed to use the sticks like tweezers around the wallet and was slowly lifting it up when . . .. Creak, slap, the outhouse door opened and shut. David had walked in oblivious to the situation. Thinking his father was sick and overcome by the fumes and was about to fall in, he grabbed his feet. Plop. Splash. The wallet lay back down onto the disgusting pile. Mark was too late with his announcement to leave Father alone and now all three stooges were now standing, staring into the dark hole. Together they attempted to retrieve the dirty wallet. After several messy tries of hooking, squeezing, and fumbling, the filthy money was pulled to the top. Then came step two. David found an old, galvanized steel washtub. The men of the family emptied the wallet of all its contents into clean water: drivers license, insurance slips, as well as all the cash. After washing it all, they decided that it needed to be dried. The adjacent, empty campsite was sunnier, and the clothesline stretched from their front porch to our cabin. With clothes pegs in hand they hung up the laundered bills and papers to dry. Since the line was not long enough David and Mark decided to lay all the extra bills on the front bumper, headlights and hood of the station wagon. Relaxing after a crazy afternoon, Father sat back in the Adirondack wooden chair where he thought he would spend the rest of the afternoon before Mom and I returned from picking up groceries in town.

Just then a car pulled in between the trees. It was some American vacationers arriving to their accommodations in the next cabin. Some explanation would be needed Father knew, but he decided to have some fun. He spun a story about needing more money for the second week of vacation and that this was his last batch of money drying. He sat back with a poker face and watched them as they began to warily unpack. After a half hour the gig was up and Father came clean with the neighbours. They were howling!

Every family has their side-splitting stories or tall tales hidden in photo books or hope chests. Now is the time to unpack the memories and laugh until it hurts to lighten the load. It melts the stress even if it's just for a short time.

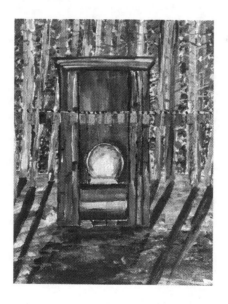

Chapter 17

WEDDING WORDS

LIFE OFTEN SEEMS TO CONSIST OF COMPARISONS AND COMPETITION. In every family it seems one child excels in school while another struggles, one is musically gifted while another is tone deaf or one is sporty and another awkward. We all fall on a spectrum of categories. My father, being the last child born to a mother of forty-three years of age, often found himself at the low end of the scale on most categories.

"Why can't you spell like your brother?" one teacher sputtered when Lyndon sat down after only one round of the spelling bee in the one room schoolhouse.

"Your older sister would have read two books and you have only finished the first paragraph," another teacher stated the next year. As well as not being gifted academically, he could not sing a note, and sports was not his forte. Cruel put-downs by adults and children alike may drive many kids to violence or depression, however, for my father, these experiences developed in him an ability to care for the underdog and have compassion for the forgotten.

For as long as I can remember my father picked up hitchhikers. He had been a hitchhiker once travelling from Truro, Nova Scotia, to Toronto, Ontario, in search of work. Through grit and determination, he had found work after arriving and he was therefore, willing to help any stranger: whether it be a hitchhiker needing a ride, a stranger needing a day's work, or a foreign professor needing a place to stay. If Father brought someone in the car, or to our home, it was my job to make them feel welcome. I was the one to collect the paint or tools for the makeshift work that Father would assign people needing money, or I was to be the conversationalist. Strangers from off the bus often stayed in our home as an in-between place until they could get settled. Seeing this obvious love for people would affect me deeply.

I can now clearly see the greatest lesson he ever preached was through his actions on my wedding day. My father stroked the veil back in place as the gentle wind tried to reveal my smiling face. Today I would leave Mother and Father and cling to my husband, but the leaving was breaking his heart as he held the car door open. My mother and her mother, Nana, (who suffered with dementia), slipped into the back seats. My father looked over at me as he started the car and I could see he was about to say something, but his eyes said it all. He was proud of me and he loved me. Sun streamed through the glass etched window kissing my cheek as my father let go of my arm at the altar and I stood beside this new man who would vow to take me and love me unconditionally as my father had. The transfer was bittersweet as my father was my hero, and now my prince charming would take his place. The day melted like cotton candy, sweet and almost gone too fast. It was time for the speeches. I was his only little girl and on this day his speech would be the crescendo of all the feelings and love I knew we had shared which would now be put into words. I thought this was my blessing, his words, a treasured gift wrapped in bow.

"The father of the bride will say a few words," the master of ceremonies introduced. No one stood. Awkward silence lingered while the master of ceremonies pointed in the direction of my mother. She stood in her mint green dress dignified and beautiful and spoke something, but I barely heard a word. Where was my father? Why wasn't he here? Moments of self pity stung like chewed sour candy I couldn't swallow. How could my father miss the most important moment of my life? Where was he? The weakening clapping slowed as my mother sat. The evening washed away, and I was whisked to Europe, a continent away, with my new husband.

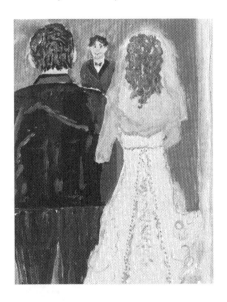

— ❄ —

As I ferry my dad around now and I drive past the wedding hall where I had sat twenty-five years ago waiting for my dad's speech, I reflect. I learned many months after my wedding why he was not there. Graciously he volunteered to take his mother-in-law, Nana with dementia, back to the nursing home. He knew that in the evening she would have become agitated and would probably cause a scene. I now understand. Evenings present challenges and are difficult for people with this sickness. She might embarrass herself or taint the evening for me, yet he wanted to give her time to enjoy the wedding meal but not disturb my reception. He figured he would have enough time to drive her back to the nursing home and be back in time for his speech.

His life was his speech and now I also choose to love and be as thoughtful to him as he was to his mother-in-law. I want to display the same tenderness and thoughtfulness which he lived. Life is not about how bright or gifted you are, but about how brightly the love of Jesus shines through you.

Chapter 18

FALL LEASHES AND RESTRAINTS!

"HELP!" SCREECHED A FOUR-YEAR-OLD BROTHER AS HIS MOTHER teetered off the top step which led to a basement with cement flooring. My father, who was puttering on old vacuums and tinkering with broken motors, leapt across the room kangaroo style to catch his top-heavy pregnant wife. The yell, the leap, the catch, probably saved my life as she slammed into his strong loving arms instead of the thud of the floor.

Today, as every day, I turn the key and unlatch the door. With his heart rate so high and his increasing fragility, I steel myself for what I might see at the bottom of the steps. I usually head to the piano and flip up the old wooden lid. After turning to a favourite hymn, I play loudly. It is my calling card. He complains about the walls in his upstairs bedroom shaking, but I am his alarm clock and I know that secretly he likes the wake-up music. It is our routine. I normally would proceed up the old brown shag carpeted steps to his bedroom door on the left, knock, and announce what day of the week it is and what the agenda will be. But today, when I entered the house, the movie clip from the <u>Wizard of Oz</u> where the witch's feet are sticking out from under the collapsed house meets me in living color.

I was not there to catch my father falling down the stairs as he had caught me 50 years before. My father's slippered feet were sticking out from behind the sliding door at the bottom of the main level stairs beside the family piano. Thoughts race like rats to dark sewage water. *Has he had a heart attack? Is he dead? Did he break something?*

"Dad?" I scurry, dropping purse, bag, and keys to uncover which train of thought would be our reality.

"Is it you?" I hear a weak defeated voice. "Is it you?" he repeats.

Half of my fears are tamped down like a whack-a-mole game, but other questions are popping up.

"Are you ok?" I scrunch down beside him.

"My arm—I think it is broken."

"What happened?" Asking an Alzheimer's patient that question is like asking a toddler a calculus question. I try, like a crime scene investigator, to deduce the event that led to this.

"I don't know," he stammers. "I think I was up there," he points with his uninjured arm toward the top of the stairs. He hollers as he tries to maneuver himself towards me. "I can't move. I can't sit up." After several minutes I hoist him to a sitting position only to have him flop back down. We lie on the floor together.

This was the time for a heart to heart. "You know, soon you might have to go into a home. Someone is usually here most of the time but not every single minute is covered."

"I just fell,' he states stubbornly. "Get me up!"

"I can't until Spencer comes." I sigh.

My nineteen-year-old, gym dedicated son dead lifted his Grampy up off the carpet and half carries the dead-weighted broken body through the kitchen, out the door, down the outside porch steps, and into the passenger side of the family car.

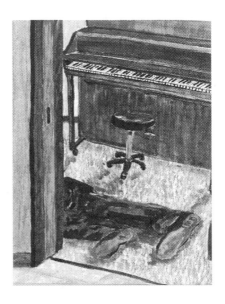

No one thinks about doctors, nurses, and hospitals until you are engulfed behind the doors in the emergency wing. Waiting in the breeze way for x-rays, then more waiting for other tests, and a ride on a stretcher to another waiting area are all parts of the journey. Nurses whisper while you wait. Technicians wheel others while you wait. After 15 hours, he was admitted with a chipped shoulder blade and unbeknownst to us, a pneumonia pronouncement. When it is time for bed for me a heavenly cloud swallows me, but not so for Dad in the hospital.

The second night when we explained that he had to stay for the medicine to be administered, fear and panic set in. The I.V. was disastrous. He looked like a drug user of 20 years, pocked with puncture holes where they had tried and failed to find fresh healthy veins. But more was to come.

Most of us have memories of dogs pulling on leashes in yards barking wildly. Knowing that, I never thought I would choose, as a young mom, to buy a leash or child harness for my child to walk along beside me. Usually when I went to the mall with all three children, I was very focused on what needed to be purchased with the quickest exit route planned. However, one day while taking a short cut through the clothing section of Walmart to the food section, I saw some women's shirts for sale on a high double rack. I momentarily stopped to flip through the sale items. My older two children stood waiting but my third was wandering off with a stranger speaking to him quietly. When I looked down and saw the littlest being enticed away, I yelled, "Hey! That's my kid!" Evan stopped and turned, and the man continued quickly away. I ran and swooped up my child into a fierce hug and an overflow of tears streaked down my face. I rarely went shopping after that. When I finally did, it was with the new harness I had purchased. It was snuggly secured on my youngest child's chest connected to my waist and the other two held each of my hands. Young women would scowl at me, but I understood the dangers of not using a harness for restraint and control.

Leashes are used for dogs, harnesses for keeping children close, but restraints for the elderly was something I hadn't thought through before. A voice on the line from the hospital brought me back to awareness, "The night nurse left a message for you," the flat-voiced day nurse stated, "Your dad was so agitated and aggressive last night, they had to put him in restraints." Her statement was like a weather channel warning flashing across my screen during my favorite TV show. You knew that what was coming was bad but hoped it might not be nearly as bad as predicted. I drove to the hospital tucking that information into my mental pocket like putting a dirty Kleenex in my jeans, yucky and out of sight. I walked into the pea green room, not sure what I expected to see. The crazed man glared through me and that Kleenexed information became like chewed gum in my hair. Just like trying to remove gum from one's hair, I pulled at the realization of the true storm that I was encountering. Few memories are as burned into my soul as this one. Dad lurched at me like a chained dog. Panicking I stopped and stared.

His fiery eyes pleaded and raged simultaneously. "You have got to get me out of here. They are all crazy. They are poisoning me." All the while he was heaving against the straps. Somehow, he sensed my terror and huskily grovelled to entice me to come closer within the range of his leash. "They are in it together. The doctors hurt the nurses and there is yelling in here. I can't stay here! They have locked me down!! You have got to get me out of here!!!" His voice was rising with each statement. He reefed and chafed against the rough blue ankle restraints and the midriff tie down.

Jesus, I prayed. *I cannot understand, but You do. You are God and you allowed cruel men to restrain you with nails to be my dad's Saviour-my Saviour too. You understand he is human and diseased while you are perfect and yet you died restrained to ultimately free us and save us.* The old tattered Bible story book my dad read to me as a child flipped instantaneously in my mind to the picture of Jesus on the ground being nailed to the cross in that moment. I knew Jesus took on the sin and sickness of mankind but seeing the ravages of this disease on a broken sinful man, my dad, was disturbing. My eyes blinked back the moment and I swallowed the tears like a walled dam. *I have to be strong,* I thought, as my body quivered involuntarily. The mental interaction with the Divine had calmed me. *It is alright. The doctors and staff are trying to keep everyone safe.* And then my mind waffled. *Yeah, right!* The rebuttal interjected itself into my inner dialogue, but I dared not look at the nurses with the same judgment with which young women had regarded me in the mall when I had walked along with my harnessed toddler.

"But God, dear God, this is brutal!" It is brutal to see a man so distressed. It was surreal; a lurching man chained to a bed asking

for his freedom. I somehow held together a stoic, mannequin face until I could escape to the hall, then finally out to my car where I collapsed like ruins after flooding. In my watery state, I blubbered over the phone to my brother in Vancouver about the storm I had lived through. His calming voice quoted a few lines from a poem:

Do not go gentle into that good night,
Old age should burn and rave at close of day;
Rage, rage against the dying of the light.[6]
"It is ok for Dad to rage. He is struggling to live. It's ok for you to cry," he comforted.

A torrent inside me let go and I sobbed uncontrollably while he simply breathed miles away from the storm. I whimpered until there was nothing left to do. I sucked in the stale air in the dark car and drove home.

On day three of the week-long hospital stay I arrived ten minutes too late. Blood and water were on the floor, and he was in his bed. The male nurse met me before I stepped in. "Your dad has fallen. He got out of the chair, even with the dinner tray attachment in front of him and fell. There are no broken bones, just a scraped elbow." I conceded in my mind that restraints are sometimes necessary no matter how awful they seem.

Jesus nails of willing restraints bought our freedom. Dad's restraints keep him safe on planet earth a little longer until he is safe in the arms of our resurrected Jesus. There Dad will be free to run, fly and worship.

---

6   Poem "Do not Go Gentle in that Dark Night" Dylan Thomas - 1914-1953

Chapter 19

HELP! I AM NOT A NURSE

MOTHER THERESA AND FLORENCE NIGHTINGALE ARE NAMES THAT are synonymous with kindness, gentleness, and extreme compassion. I am a teacher. I only thought of two professions for women as a young girl: teaching and nursing. I rarely was sick and don't really have patience with those who are. Teaching is my profession. Using objects, excitement, and even drama to explain the sound that 'p' makes, or dramatizing the French revolution is my preferred career. I taught in a private school for five years before embarking on the journey to homeschool my sons for the span of the next 15 years. If my student, my child was sick, well, that just meant I would carry the books to his room and read aloud to him. If he was *really* sick, he could sleep through class. Sickness, from my experience and definition, is only a blimp until health returns and normalcy begins the next day. However, with Alzheimer's, the sickness begins and only ends when death comes.

After leaving the hospital with Dad, the doctor's words rang repeatedly in my ears. "He needs 24-hour care. He can never be left alone; never, not even one hour." Time became the enemy, life became boxes. I was free spirited and was almost an empty nester, gaining new wings to fly, and hoping for new adventures to journey. My thoughts flew apart like a shot gun blast. I felt dead. I felt trapped.

Carefully, my friend and I helped push him up the three back steps of his home. My new prison, was the house I had grown up in. After my shift, I rushed home and jumped onto Facebook and wrote:

I know God's ways are good and I know eventually the government will try to or encourage us to euthanize ourselves or our loved ones instead of caring for them. I struggle with this new path that I am called to travel because I do know right from wrong, and though euthanizing him never crossed my mind, neither did I think I would need to become his fulltime caregiver.

For three years my father had been my constant morning companion. I took him with me to Ladies' Bible studies, social functions, antique stores, and Wendy's every Wednesday for lunch. Three years ago, I had internally fought to give up those 15 hours a week to caregiving, but now we had a routine and things were comfortable. He had been with me while gardening and doing odd jobs, just like a mother includes her child while still accomplishing the tasks at hand. Now things would be different. Fewer day trips, fun, and people would be traded for confinement, care, and entrapment with longer hours. I wrestled with this. How would he and I handle this new reality, full daytime care?

"I don't want to eat."

"Don't force me to eat."

"I'm not hungry."

Seriously, had I slipped and hit my head and returned twenty years to mothering a baby?

Dad did not want to eat. "When you don't eat, you feel weak, and lousy. Then you feel dizzy, and you fall. The more you sleep and don't eat or move, the more incapacitated you get," I spouted this logic to my dad. Reasoning does not work on toddlers, and it doesn't work with dementia patients. I, as the nurse, would have to develop new tactics. How were my brother and I going to get this man to eat?

I scheduled caretakers to come in to help with a few of the hours. My brother always had to leave in the morning before I could arrive after my early morning job of teaching English online. He had been staying home later in the mornings putting his job at risk because he felt he must ensure that Dad had eaten something and taken his medicine. Workers from the community services came to alleviate that time of stress. They would spend the hour and a half to help him get into a morning routine so Mark did not have to rush him. They would get him up and dressed and then help him down the stairs to the table to begin the coaxing or distracting methods to ensure that some food was ingested with the pills.

Personal support workers are so needed and helpful, but they are exactly that, personal. Since they do not work in a manufacturing company, they often are late because the clients previous to your scheduled time have needed extra time or emergencies had arisen. The company that hired them would often fail to have people ready to fill in for them if they were sick or they would leave no time in the schedule between the clients for the workers to travel and navigate throughout the city. When they were there for the time they were scheduled, they were very supportive, and it was helpful. Nursing embodies compassion and patience. I would have to learn this new art form.

My dad, being proud and stubborn, refused to let the personal support workers help him into the bath.

"Why don't you just let them help you?" I argued with him one afternoon. That was when I realized that he had gone two months without a shower, and no one was able to coax him into the tub. Something needed to be done and I set my resolve to do it. Two hours later, with dignity intact, five soaked towels and a drenched, exhausted old man, the deed was done; it was not done well or gracefully but the task was completed. As a daughter I could never have envisioned having to attempt such a difficult undertaking. My brother realized that he would have to take that role on as I could not repeat the process and the PSW's had not been successful. Lifting, lowering, buttoning, assisting, that was nursing. I can not say I do these tasks always with patience or finesse, but my heart is slowly melting with more kindness like the butter on our weekly Wendy's baked potato.

Sometimes my husband hears me sigh as I leave my home for my daily new 8-hour shift of caring for Dad. I have a pep talk with myself and a serious talk with the Lord on the drive over. It helps me enter his home ready to bring love and joy through my care. Slowly, I am creatively coming up with new ideas of things to do to occupy our time. When he naps, I read books that I have never taken the time to read. I find pleasure in the daily routine. We sort nuts and bolts, do simple puzzles, I read to him, and play the piano for him. The advice of taking it one day at a time is the only way to travel this road of care.

Chapter 20

SPOT THE DIFFERENCES

<u>Spot the Difference</u> activity books teach kids to observe and notice small differences. Our heads turn when someone has a flattened nose or walks with a limp. We try not to stare but we notice it. If you are in a sea of purple people, you would notice the blue person. If you were in Lilliput[7] you would notice the lone giant. Differences are a part of life.

I grew up in a white community knowing of other cultures but not experiencing them. I never thought of my dad as prejudiced, but sometimes with his Alzheimer's mind, he would step back in time to Nova Scotia, and he'd begin a story with "at 'N' Hill". I would shut him down.

"We don't talk that way. That is inappropriate to even say." I would stifle the memory or refuse to let his story continue. Was he a racist deep down? I did not want to know.

Who or what you think is a direct reflection of your personal history and present experience. Then and there I decided to introduce my family to other cultures. My husband and I became a student house when our boys were teens. We have eaten dinner with Muslims from Saudi Arabia, a boy from Spain, an older teen from Brazil, and

---

[7]   Dr. Jonathan Swift, 1727, Gulliver's Travels

another from China who turned out to be not your stereotypical studious student. We learned about the peoples of our world. No one can say people are all the same because culture, tradition, and the arts make each race unique. I agree with this message from one of Dr. Seuss' books, *Horton Hears a Who.* "A person's is a person, no matter how small!"[8] which can be interpreted to mean a person is a person no matter what race. Though we may be very different in colour and culture, we are all of equal value because God made every person in His image.

One day, after reading a short story to my dad about a poor boy in England who worked in the mines and the difficulties their family encountered, a monologue of my dad's life ensued.

"I knew people back in Nova Scotia who worked in the mines," he began. "Our family was poor too. During the depression, Papa lost his job, but we survived." My dad always referred to his dad as Papa. He continued, "Mama managed to make large pots of veggie stew for our family. The carrots were stubby and the potatoes less plentiful considering the acreage. Papa was a short, serious man who tried to supplement the family income through the rented farmland." The far distant memories of this eighty-year-old morphed him back into a boy of eight. I could envision the story as he brought living colour to the old scenes. "I travelled in the old horse drawn wagon into town with Papa on market days. We stood there calling out prices but not many people had the money to purchase the goods we brought. We only sold a small percentage of the produce we had taken to sell. People just could not afford it. Piling all the vegetables back into the wagon, we headed back home."

Growing up I knew my father as a very generous man, and I

---

[8]   Horton Hears a Who. Dr Seuss

guessed that I was about to learn about the roots of how that quality developed. My dad's voice brought me back into his script.

"There was a definite separation of who lived where and with whom. The blacks lived on 'N'-Hill." I cringed as he said it; but this time I let him continue as there was no malicious intent in his voice when he spoke those words, just a factual recounting of his memories.

"'Lyndon, we can't possibly use all this food. It will go to waste. They have less than we do,' my papa stated matter-of-factly. So, Papa turned the wagon left toward 'N'- Hill."

My dad, sitting in the peach-coloured living room chair in Ontario, looked through me as though he could see the black folks of Nova Scotia watching suspiciously through their broken shuttered windows. He continued, "Papa stepped down from the wagon and knocked on the first paint peeling door with some vegetables in hand. The large black woman was wary at first, but she smiled and received the vegetables from my papa, a white man. We extended food and compassion, and many received what Papa and I brought."

'N'-Hill for my dad was synonymous with generosity. It was here that cultural barriers were crossed, and kindness was practiced in a time and in a province when that was not the norm.

My dad wrapped up the story, "From then on, any unsold produce was shared with those on the 'Hill' who definitely had less than we white folks did. Black people came out of their shacks for the remainder of the harvest on market day when they heard the wagon wheels of the MacBain food cart driven by the short man with a big heart, my papa," Dad's story ended abruptly.

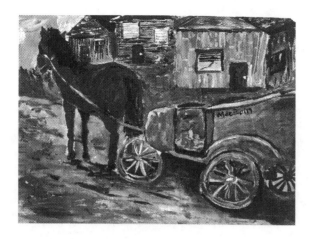

My eyes filled as the story concluded, realizing that I had got stuck on the political incorrectness of words even though love and kindness was cloaked in crude vocabulary. I would leave that afternoon and a woman of African descent would arrive from social services to care for my dad. Her toothy smile was big and her size looming as she shook my dad's hand for the first time in this role to him.

"Remember me? You drove me on the bus to my first job after I arrived in Canada. I still remember your welcoming smile which calmed me as you talked and cajoled with all the passengers," she reminisced and addressed my dad.

He smiled, blankly pretending to remember.

"Well, it is good to see you," she stated realizing that he did not know her. She would return the kindness and become his favourite Personal Support Worker in the days ahead. The people of all nations were coming to him and although it was obvious most of them loved what they did, it was not a job many could remain in because of a variety of work salary issues. The wonderful black woman with whom he had come to enjoy visiting also left her employment.

A flood of new people came. The change of routine and unfamiliar faces wreaked havoc on my aging dad with Alzheimer's.

As children, we accept change and when my father was a boy, he did too. My father, who lived through the depression as a youngster, related how his mama decided to take in a Jewish baby that she found left on her wood pile one spring morning.

The doctor reminded her that she already had enough mouths to feed. "Why should you take in some Jewish girl's cast away child?" the doctor challenged.

She explained that every child deserved a loving home, food, and shelter. Dad's mama demonstrated generosity when their family took that baby in as their own. My father loved his new adopted brother although his presence would stretch the meager resources and space in their home.

Now Dad's space as an elderly man was being invaded. Men from India and the Middle East came for the Friday night shifts. Women from Latin America and Africa came in the afternoon to bathe and help him. Whether it was simply the sea of changing faces, or sexes, or heavy accents which he could not decode, his frustration rose. Often people from other places are soft spoken which added to the stress of my father because of decreased hearing. These struggles worked in tandem to reveal a yelling, rude man who often appeared racist.

"Why are you here?" I heard him roar at a quiet spoken Hispanic woman as I was shutting the screen door, leaving an hour early from my time with him. "I don't need you here, go back to your own country," he continued as I walked sadly to my car. Sometimes the Personal Support Workers could calm him down and at other times it would escalate into threats of calling the police on them. Recognizing that he wasn't getting his way, he began and continued to say inappropriate or degrading things to try to get them to leave. Many of these outbursts were nasty verbal jabs. My brother and I found ourselves often apologizing for these incidences when we knew of them. Disease is not an excuse for that, and embarrassment became part of the humiliation price we paid for the careless words that spewed out of his mouth in his desire to control his surroundings.

I am not surprised that people from various other nations gravitate to jobs involving caring for the elderly because I believe that most other cultures view the older generation with respect and as having value even though their bodies and minds may deteriorate. Much to our shame in the US and Canada, we are moving to an attitude of simply wanting to rid ourselves of the elderly by shutting them away or euthanizing them.

The many Personal Support Workers we encountered were kind and capable. They were gracious even when difficult situations arose. These workers were coming in from other nations and caring wonderfully for my dad and others like him who are sometimes belligerent, who speak rudely and who act inappropriately. I am so grateful to all who enter this profession to care for the forgotten, the difficult, the stubborn old people who battle their own minds, people with dementia.

Chapter 21

YOU FORGOT MY NAME

TODAY HE FORGOT MY NAME. THOUGHTS CRASHED TOGETHER LIKE waves against a cliff.

I've been here for four years. The next wave crests; *35-40 hours a week away from my home, my family, caring for you.* The highest wave mounts; *you don't know my name!* I stay silent, but the deafening thoughts roar through my stubborn heart. *No Dad, I'm not telling you my name; you will remember it.* I mentally push back. *I am your only daughter. My dreams, my aspirations, and my life have been majorly interrupted and you don't even know my name!* Yes, I know these thoughts are selfish, so my better side rises to argue. However, this is real! It cannot be happening to me, and an undertow of thinking threatens. Then I see something behind his eyes, as though looking into his inner mind. I visualize cog wheels turning slowly past the notches of memory unable to lock in on my name. He is frustrated as he tries to introduce me to the case worker, and I sit silent for another moment not wanting to fill in the blank. I wait. But then the waves of anger wash away and I fill the empty, awkward space for Dad. "I am Carolyn. Thanks for taking care of my dad today." The storm on the sea of my mind calms.

This lack of memory is what many call a senior's moment. He can't pick a name, a word, or an idea out of the file folder of words stacked in his brain. That drawer did not open for him at that moment. Before the personal support worker finishes packing up, he asks me to get his tea using my name as though he had never struggled to remember it. The file drawer opened. I sigh at my selfishness and yet I expect that in future days he may be permanently locked out of that file folder which holds my name. Memories of me or even the acknowledgement of my existence may become closed to him forever, but not today. One day I may face the genuine words, *"Who are you? You look familiar, but do I know you?"*

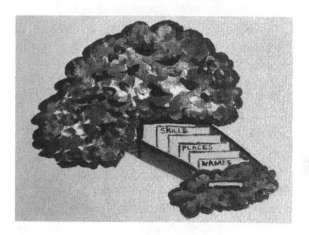

While he slept that day quietly in his room, I listen to a Christian talk radio station to soothe my soul and to my surprise it was a bittersweet story about marriage and dementia. My thoughts ran toward the idea of how spouses would handle this horrible disease. Many have experienced the love of their life forgetting who they are. I try to imagine years of marriage forgotten. What if my lover, my best friend, and partner did not recognize who I was? It is unfathomable to imagine these memories stolen. Unfortunately it is part of the breaking down of the disease and destruction of the mind.

Now that I was totally depressed, the radio announcer's words interrupted my negative mood. "I want to share a story that may bless some of you going through difficult times with a loved one with dementia." She continued in a description of an elderly woman's pain as her husband of many years forgot who she was. The woman made a choice to honour her vows for better or for worse and care lovingly for him. Most stories I had listened to like this, ended with the man finding another woman in the nursing home or the man treating his wife, whom he didn't now know or recognize, cruelly, but this story would be one of beauty from ashes, one full of redemptive qualities. Tears trickled down my cheeks as I envisioned walking that horrible road between spouses and yet tears of joy would be coming as the Christian broadcaster continued her story. The woman's caring kindness and loving persistence attracted the elderly man back. One day, out of the blue, unable to even remember her as his wife or even her name, he asked if she would marry him. She gladly accepted and she is enjoying the fact that she could marry the same man twice in one lifetime. Her joy was evident instead of bitterness for the loss as it was shared by the host through the airwaves. Though not all stories have happy endings this unusual story was a beautiful one I needed to hear that day.

Names are extremely important! Whenever a human is referred to as a number, they are depersonalized.

"Number 56, please come forward. It is your turn at the government license office."

"Number 47, the doctor will see you now."

But one of the worst times in history, where the ultimate dehumanization occurred was when the Jewish people were tattooed with numbers and later disposed of in horrible ways. We are not meant to be numbers or treated as such. A name has meaning, and it is associated with the person you love.

I vowed that even if he forgot my name, Carolyn which means song or joy, or who I was, I would not become indifferent to him.

Like many, I wonder at how I will truly handle this lose of memory but this scripture rips through my memory.

"See I have engraved (or tattooed) you on the palms of my hands."[9]

Jesus knows the horrible things that men did to human beings in those concentration camps, as well as the awful things disease does to minds, but he never forgets us. He knows our thoughts, our rising up, our going out, and he knows our names. We are figuratively tattooed on his hands. His love for us is unconditional. God will never forget me, and God will never forget Dad even if the connection on earth between us disconnects. It will be extremely hard to traverse that road of forgetfulness together, but every person needs to be treated with kindness even if they don't recognize the person who is caring for them.

Alzheimer's is cruel and yet for now, Dad does know who I am. It is hard to focus on the present, but I take joy in the fact that he knows who I am today. I will not worry about tomorrow.

---

[9]   Isaiah 49:16 A New International Version.

Chapter 22

INCARCERATION

My brother Mark's voice on the other end of the phone line paused, and then in staccato sentences he relayed the message of the long awaited, dreaded call from a nursing home.

"There's a bed."

"I'm not ready."

"Let's say no."

Mark had shouldered most of the weight of care as he lived with Dad. The morning procedures, the supper routines, and the bedtime rituals were all woven into his life. I was there for much of the daytime but I had the help of a paid friend and few hours of weekly community help. By this point, people knew when to come and go. Routines of piano playing, reading, Uno games, and outings were running like the melody of a Beethoven's sonata. Sometimes notes however, were misplaced or a page from the routine fell off the piano ledge, but overall it was working. Just two weeks before that call my brother had slipped across to his own house on a Saturday afternoon to try to get some repairs done thinking that our dad was in a comfortable afternoon nap. Then he a got a different call.

"We are just letting you know that we just brought your dad in by ambulance," the lady on the other end of the line announced.

Only a half hour had slipped past but Dad who had woken, felt chest pain, called out, and not receiving a response dialed 911. We knew we were fighting a battle on two fronts: the slowing heart and the dementia. After retrieving him from the hospital, we increased his heart medications to the full amount prescribed by the doctor even though that might increase his risk of falling. The delicate balance of his safety, managing pain, and twenty-four-hour care was taking its toll on us, even though neither my brother or I wanted to admit it.

"We have to take the nursing home placement," I responded to the quietness on the other end of the line after Mark's announcement. "If we turn it down, we will be at the bottom of the waiting list and it may be months before we can move him in."

"The timing is wrong," came his terse response. He breathed deeply and plunged on, "We have so much to do to get his house ready to rent or sell. And he is doing okay, right now."

Caregiving had become my single brother's whole world. This would be like a death to him, and I struggled with the guilt as well. I cringed. We were paralyzed. Whenever I had spoken to Dad about his care, he had always responded with a snide remark. "Why would I need to go to a nursing home?"

When one is young, parents encourage, cajole, and maybe even force their child to go to places like camp. It often depended on the personality of the child, but the parents know their child would have a wonderful time with great memories and new friends. However, this placement could not be compared to sending a child off to camp. There was no returning home. In my thinking, by dropping him off into a nursing home, there would be no good memories for him there. If this truly was what God wanted for our elderly parent, I did not feel it. But I pushed on. We had to say yes to the home. I took my youngest son, eighteen, at the time, to his Grampy's house to help transport some personal belongings: his furniture, a painting, and some clothes. To accomplish this task without questions, I asked the Personal Support Worker to distract my dad with tea and crumpets in the kitchen. All the while Evan stole about the house behind closed doors sneaking the things into my waiting van for transport to the nursing home. How deceitful we were! How wrong we felt! I could only imagine my dad's look of disbelief and betrayal if he could see through the walls of his very own house at the shenanigans happening all around him.

We were instructed that setting up his room ahead of time was paramount to the success of moving in a resistant resident. Evan and I walked into the nursing home. I steeled myself that the entire plan may backfire, but in that moment, the present and a past memory collided. I saw myself carrying a sleeping bag to a cabin on a picturesque lakefront with a nervous boy ladened with one week's worth of clothes and toiletries beside me wondering why his mother was making him go. The screen play was interrupted as a man in the hall hollered profanity and Dad's new roommate grunted about the dead man that used to live in the other half of the room. We unpacked Dad's belongings. I involuntarily shook. My grown son's eyes were that of the little boy by the lake but much more terrified and saddened. This was not a room by the lake. This was a prison cell. Slowly, I instructed him to hang up Grampy's clothes in the closet while I busied myself unpacking the few other trinkets to place on a prefabricated, wooden nightstand. We brought in his other few belongings and his painting. The single bed, not as crude as a camp bunkbed, was tiny for a grown man. Emotions swallowed us both up. We walk back through the hallway of drooling empty-eyed skin-covered ghosts reaching to touch us. Evan rushed and passed me through the locked exit punching in the code to get out. I wanted to run too but I forced myself to walk to the car stifling the tears, trying to be strong. "What was I doing?"

Struggling and quiet, I started the car. My son stared out the passenger window, "Mom, what you are doing is wrong!" It felt like a judgmental pronouncement.

Tears rushed down my face like a car wash, but I did not feel clean. This was a nightmare, and tomorrow I would take my dad to jail. I barely slept, and I knew my brother had not slept for the last four nights since the call. We knew that this was Dad's last night watching a crackling fire and a rerun of "Gun Smoke" on his own TV in his own home. Choosing not to inform him felt like treason.

Mark drove up the next morning with Dad in the car and I followed in my car. I knew my brother desperately did not want to do this. My son's words were fresh in my head. Thankfully my husband was giving me space without pressure. Yet I felt like I was in a pressure cooker. I was the only one who was pushing us to follow through on the decision. I drove alone and flipped on the Christian radio station 99.9 Grace FM. The song, "God help me" by Plumb had just started to play. I had tried to remember this song for the past two weeks and could not remember the title but here and now the words blared in my ears.

"There is a wrestling in my heart and my mind.
A disturbance and a tension I cannot seem to drive,
And if I'm honest, there's quite a bit of fear,
To sit here in this silence and really hear You.
What will you ask of me?"[10]

The song continues with words begging God to help me move, help me see, and help me go forward. It expressed sentiments of barely breathing and yet knowing that God would help. The radio station simply played the songs of choice in a queue but for me that was God reaching down and holding me steady to the decision that I had made. The song ended on the final turn into the nursing home. God's presence had wrapped me up, not like a warm fuzzy blanket, but there was a sense of knowing that God would go with all of us through this deep water. As we exited the cars, I remembered that I had promised my brother that if Dad did not settle, we would bring him back home. I had friends praying that Lyndon would settle and we would have clear direction that what we were doing was the right thing. Robotically, I stuffed down the memory of Dad in the hospital a year before in

---

[10]   *"God Help Me"* by Plumb (Tiffany Arbuckle Lee)

restraints fighting like a mad dog to be free. We would have to try. I pretended this to be a camp adventure and Dad would be okay, yet I feared the worst. Murders happened in nursing homes. I knew personally of a friend whose parent had been pushed by a resident and later died from head injuries. "*God, this is not camp*," my mind shouted.

Dad was quiet. My brother told him a half truth. "We are going here to get your swelling feet checked. The doctors and nurses will help you. You may have to stay for a few days." He shuffled along to his room and sat in his own faded, peach-coloured wing-backed chair. No comment was made about his favorite painting on the wall. He just looked out the window to the squared courtyard where winter's remains left a gloomy colour which enveloped us all.

Mark and I proceeded to sign documents discussing medicine and food likes and dislikes as though the man was not even there. There was no reaction. It was as though Dad had flat lined into this new lifeless reality. I encouraged my brother to go back to work. I knew the strain and the guilt was about to take over his face which would then alert Dad to what was truly happening. At lunch, I was seated at a table with a fish aquarium directly across from me. The dull-coloured fish in the tank was slowly sinking to the bottom. It was floating up, up, and then slipping down struggling ever so slightly but obviously dying. I blinked and swallowed the tears. I sat still, trying to grapple with death, trying to process the entrapment, trying to understand the not getting out. I was overwhelmed by guilt for putting him here.

My dad sat to my left. Directly across from him at the next table was a man being spoon feed by a hovering nurse. The food was dribbling down the side of his face and I could see my dad trying to process this. He was staring. What did he see, his fate? Did he see the man in the other chair being stuffed to death as his future? All living things here died. Suddenly, I saw it in my dad's eyes. There was a bit of fear and a bit of recognition. He turned to watch the fish. Did he see that he was in a fishbowl going down to the bottom of the tank? Slowly the struggling fish succumbed. Its life ebbed away;

it floated upside down toward the top. Everything crossed his face all at once as he turned to me. He knew. I knew. Death was here. Death would come. He motioned with his head toward the other man and his voice lowered and he stammered, "Don't feed me like that. Don't ever feed me like that." Then his gaze returned to the freshly floating dead fish.

We finished up lunch. There was no anger. I had waited for the anger. Bringing him here I thought would bring him into full blown rage or maybe into fight mode. But many people had given their time to pray and were asking God to give us all peace of mind. This was the acid test. Would we be taking him back home or would he settle? The floating fish faded. Lunch morphed into an afternoon of nurses and people. I left just before dinner. He asked if I would be back to take him home that night. I left ensuring him that I would be back tomorrow.

Untangling false or real guilt occupied my mind for the first two weeks. But I was committed to going daily to aid in the transition. It had been my routine to care for him so to simply hand it over to complete strangers seemed like abandonment. What would the new normal be like? On the second day, I sat with Dad in a hymn sing. Maybe there could be joy found here and maybe even hope.

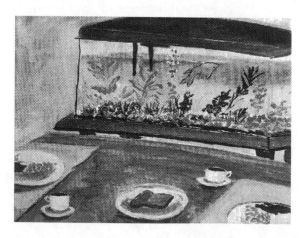

Chapter 23

A NEW NORMAL

Some caregivers are so worn out by the time a placement comes that they drop off and drive away. Their journey had been so taxing or their personal lives so neglected that this is their relief. However, my brother and I had supported one another and had others come alongside of us so we could keep going with regular visits and involvement. As I anticipated this new stage, I wondered what my new normal would be like. What would be his? My planned daily visits were too long at first because the guilt was pushing me like a tractor trailer speeding down a mountain highway. If I made the wrong decision to slam on the brakes, visit less, I might jackknife like a truck drivers wishing he had handled the conditions of the road differently. I had to navigate this new road with much thought. For each person it is difficult and challenging deciding when and how often to visit. Others with loved ones in nursing homes may have suggestions, but no judgment should be passed by anyone as each must figure out the road alone. It is terribly hard to let go and be there regularly. Finally, I decided to go most weekdays for a few hours to help him get to an activity or read to him or just take him out into the courtyard where the magnolia trees promised to blossom.

One day when I arrived, the activities-coordinator was pushing four square dinner tables together and I joined in to help because the workers treated me as one of the volunteer staff. The cheery woman, Norma, with an encouraging smile and gentle touch wheeled each participant up to the table for the game. From her cart she pulled a red rubber dodge ball and explained the activity. Memories meshed. I had played four-square in grade school with a ball like that, dodge ball in high school, and played on my driveway with my own young sons with that same type of ball. What would she do with this red, herringbone patterned ball? She placed the ball calmly on the tabletop and told the residents that she wanted them to roll the ball back across the table when it came to them. Some raised their thin veined-riddled hands to the height of the tabletop. When the rolling ball veered gently toward them in slow motion, they patted the ball. The ball changed course like a sluggish golf ball circling around a hole yet missing its destination. Some residents saw the ball coming but could not raise their hands to encounter it. At first this simplistic activity seemed demeaning. It is cute to watch a baby randomly bat at an overhanging toy, but seriously, this was pathetic or so I thought. With encouragement, the ball was gently tapped by one elderly, smiling woman to the left of my dad. Then Linda, a ninety-nine-year-old lady, whose eyes had taken on a quiet determination, began to play the game. Soon the soothing words, "Good job, Jean." "Nice work, Lyndon." motivated all the participants to awaken their limbs and find joy in tabletop hand soccer. They were having fun. They were involved. There were real people. Seeing the half-lipped smiles, the short giggles, and twinkling eyes that I had viewed as dead only moments ago was lifting my heart too. I had so miscalculated the failing level of my dad's mind and physical ability.

One evening when I joined my brother for a visit, we walked down the halls towards his room. He was not there. Most dementia wards are built in a square endless loop layout so that people can continuously shuffle or walk and feel they have gone somewhere. So, we walked the building block. We rounded the track for the third time. We had peered into every room looking for him. He was not sleeping in a corner lazyboy or in a dining room chair or in the TV lounge area. Where was he?

"Don't worry," I told my brother. "There are activities in other units that the worker coordinators will take them too," I fumbled. I began to feel a little panic too after exhausting all the regular places. It was the feeling one has when you are shopping and your five-year-old isn't sitting in the stroller anymore.

'*They must know where he is*,' I mentally argued. The gentle giant male nurse responded calmly and walked us through to another area and asked if we'd checked the outer courtyard as it was a lovely warm evening. There Dad sat smiling and watching the worker, Dan. Dan was surrounded by five wheelchair-bound people and others with their walkers parked beside them. All were watching Dan as he chattered and used a hammer and saw to build a sign board in front of his captive audience. It was like watching a live tool time with Tim Allen. Mark and I pulled up chairs and joined the fun as he drilled and screwed and prattled on with the residents. They were not only fully entertained, but many of the elderly men probably felt as though they had taken part in the building of that project. Later, other artistic residents would paint the signs in bright colors. Truly there were memories to be made here, activities to fill his time, song fests to be enjoyed, and pets to be stroked on pet day. Maybe this was old people camp.

After about a month of routine, I decided that I would venture taking him out. He had grown visibly weaker upon his arrival, but that may have been a result of all the new adjustments and medicine mayhem that occurred. "God," I prayed, "please let this not be a mistake." I knew that taking him to his own home would not be wise, but he had been at my home so much over the last few years helping or watching me garden or sitting on my front porch that I decided to drive him to my home. He loved my backyard. Although we are in the city, we have seen deer come up from the back ravine in the evening periodically. The sun beat warmly on our heads as

I walked beside him that morning with his walker to the car. My mind tossed back and forth the wisdom of doing this so soon. What if I triggered something and I could not get him to go back into the nursing home at lunchtime? I pushed the threatening raincloud thought away and replaced it with the reality. It was a beautiful morning as I pulled out of the nursing home driveway. We were well within city limits passing an open area and small ravine across from the soccer field. Then we saw one deer. Then a second and a third one leapt and jumped directly in front of my car. I slowed to a stop and we watched as I breathed.

"Be still and know, know that I am God."[11] My dad loved to see wildlife and for me this was such a confirmation that yes, the triune God was with us. When we arrived, Dad chatted about seeing the deer at ten in the morning. Any feelings of sadness or disorientation dissipated with the talk of the three deer crossing. Together we worked on a project to screw the legs on a table. He dozed on the porch and woke as each of my sons and husband intermittently came out to the porch to talk with Grampy. I drove him back in time for lunch and he shuffled along beside me back into the nursing home without question or resistance.

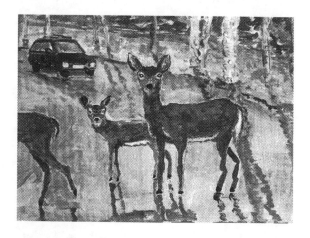

---

[11]   Psalm 46:10 King James Version

Some days at the nursing home I feel useful and even uplifted, while other days I feel as though I am walking in the halls of the living dead. At first, I saw people as fleshy corpses reaching out to me, but gradually God taught me to reach back. I would squeeze a hand, give a shoulder hug, smile, and touch them; they are real, needy people.

Over time, I noticed the small picture frames with people's faces in them sitting on the front lobby desk. When I realized they were photos of recently deceased residents, my heart filled with sadness. In the beginning I viewed this as my daily death walk into the home. At first it was depressing! But then one day that walk lit a torch in my heart. My perspective changed I would seize the day. I would gently caress a hand, speak loving words, smile warmly, and give love away to those still living another day.

"God so loved the world"[12]: tottering Edith*, emotional Sally*, speechless June*, grunting Ben*, schizophrenic John*, the lonely Bob*, and fragile Lyndon. God loved and gave his Son; I would love and give my time so that maybe some of these forgotten people could know God's love through me and believe in his Son before their picture appears on the table.

---

[12] (All the names of residents and workers have been changed.)
John 3:16 King James Version

Chapter 24

DRUGS, VIOLENCE AND SEX

I SEE MY LIFE THROUGH THE EYES OF A SANDWICHED GENERATION. My dad is the bottom slice and my son the top slice. The similarities between my dad's new nursing residence and my son's university residence is uncanny. Who will their roommates be? Will drugs, violence, or sex factor into their lives? Could my eldest son, Clayton, enter life's treadmill and not be flung off through poor choices and could my father exit life's cycle without destroying a legacy of love and gentleness as a good husband and father?

We dropped my eldest son off at the university in Hamilton at the beginning of Frosh Week. Girls in short shorts were pulling him out of the van with blaring music filling the air. His belongings were hoisted on the shoulders of jocks. His eyes were wide with excitement! This was chaos! No hug! No acknowledgement was given to us, his parents, as he was whisked away into the crowded hallways of young people, like busy ants in dimmed tunnels.

In stark contrast, my dad's drop off into the nursing home was not with the loud fanfare of the university welcoming team. It was one of deafening opposite proportions. Slumped men in wheelchairs and shuffling, sagging women filled the pristine hallways. The quiet echoes of the nurses' padded shoes along with the guttural grunts from the people in this place added to the eerie atmosphere. Dad and my son both travelled down their respective hallways to meet their new roommates.

Roommates are important. They are an integral part of the present and future which can influence you forever. My mind drifted to a roommate I had in college from New York City. She called me Carol from day one even though I introduced myself as Carolyn. This girl slept with a pool cue which she often used at night to poke and annoy me and at other times to get my attention to talk. Clayton's roommate sat on his bed surrounded by boxes like a scared mouse coming out of a hole. He seemed reserved and quiet. However, Dad's roommate was anything but quiet. From behind the half curtained off room, I heard a man with 2 personas having an entire conversation with himself. It was distressing! When I engaged in conversation with Dad's roommate later that evening, the discussion continually circled back to his escape plans from this horrible prison. Unlike furniture that is comfortable and familiar for the elderly or ratty and borrowed for a student, roommates are not furniture. They are not inanimate objects but living breathing people in your personal space and can influence you for good or for bad. Roommates of postsecondary education institutions can be depressed at times, mentally crazed during exams, or party animals out of control. So far, my son's roommate proved to be steady and was at school to study. But what about Dad's roommate?

Drugs play an enormous role in the human psyche whether you are 18 or 81. The effect of the disease on Dad's deteriorating mind required some drugs to keep the emotional equilibrium. Thankfully only infrequently at home had we encountered violent attitudes or behaviours. This was not so here for the man who would share my dad's room. He regularly talked of killing the nurse who annoyed him and other disturbing topics. After a few weeks I decided to voice my concerns to a nursing staff.

Later that evening when the phone rang, I feared the worse, but in a complete turn of events my dad had been the perpetrator.

After unscrewing the handle from a broom, he had gone into a room down the hall of a man, who hollered regularly, and hit the man with the stick. There were no videos or witnesses of the event, but the bruises were evident. Questions raced through my mind. Had my dad reacted to the negativity of his roommate and taken it out on this man or had Dad just snapped? The doctors were tweaking and toying with medications. With all the stress and changes, violence was the outcome. The phone call left me rattled. Would the family press charges? How could I judge the craziness of my dad's roommate when my dad had done worse to someone else? No one can prepare you for the endless possibilities you might encounter in life's path dealing with mental illness. No consequences came from it and the incident went away as mysteriously as it had transpired. Later that week my dad's roommate was moved to a single room. I think they feared the possible outcome of a diagnosed, unstable man bunking with an unpredictable Alzheimer's patient. The combination must have spelled trouble. We awaited a new roommate.

The telephone chirped. *"Not again,"* I thought, thinking Dad had caused some trouble, but the name that appeared across the screen's display was my son's name. He explained that the university was giving an additional week off in early fall because there had been a rash of suicides from overdoses this time last year when the weather changed. "Come home," I encouraged him. "It will be great to have you home."

Life can be hard at any stage. For youth, the stresses of their workload, parental expectations, or self devaluation can lead students to make the choice to mess with drugs to help cope or to end their lives. We do not generally consider that the elderly too, are struggling to find purpose, and in their boredom or pain want to control the only thing they can, their coming death.

Ron* was Dad's second roommate. He was a tall slim bachelor who wandered constantly and rattled the end doors at each locked corner in the boxed, square hallway maze. He rarely ate, and after the first week he shut his mouth with a quiet, but defiant determination that would seal his fate. After forty-five days of refusing sustenance, the frail bone rack of Ron* lay down for the final night. Dad slept through Ron's* passing. Life was fleeting all around him and Dad did not even know it. Things seemed to be settling in for Dad, but we were on edge as dad moved on to his third roommate.

Now it was time for some drama from the university. "My roommate's girlfriend wants to move into our room," my son stated flatly. *That quiet boy had a forward girlfriend*, I thought. The tiny room held only two single beds. It was smaller than a cheap hotel. *How awkward would that be,* my thoughts imagined. Clayton and I talked. My son and his roommate talked. After lots of discussion it was decided that none of them felt comfortable with such an awkward arrangement. The girl was soon out of the picture and all fronts went back to normal.

Dad, who had been married to my mom for 35 years until she died of cancer, and then buried his second wife after 15 years of marriage from the same disease, found himself in all kinds of compromising situations. In his confusion and exhaustion, he often slept in the closest bed he could find when he was pooped. Sometimes the woman in the room was sitting in her chair and he was in her bed snoring for the afternoon. These were innocent acts of confusion, but things were about to get more complicated.

He began to say things and act inappropriately toward the women staff and other female residents. It was devasting for me as his daughter. He was an honourable Christian husband who treated women with respect but now the filter on his mouth and self control of his hands were slipping.

Who could have ever imagined the similarities of the temptations and struggles that would hound both my young son and my aged dad? They both survived, but not without a lot of prayer from this mom and daughter.

Chapter 25

TOUCH NOT THE CAT
WITHOUT A SHIELD

IT WAS 2 AM AND WITH EYES BLURRED AND CLOTHES ON INSIDE OUT, I drove through the blackened night. I was emerging out of my sleepy state into an adrenaline rush while the blinding silent snow swirled about my car. My vehicle knew the path to the nursing home, and it travelled automatically even though its driver wasn't fully cognitive. It was not just raining in my life but snowing. That late fall afternoon, I had driven through a snowstorm to retrieve my brother, Mark, from a nearby town after a cancer surgery. Now here I was on the road heading to the nursing home in the middle of the night.

It seemed like lately whenever the phone rang and the name of the nursing home appeared on its display, something was amiss. The phone rang at 1:45 am, rousing me from sleep, I panicked; this was not a call from the home, but one from my brother in Vancouver. "You need to go now to the nursing home. Mark is heading there because Dad is kicking down doors, but Mark doesn't want you to be there. But I think," David said emphatically, "you need to go!"

Who knows what sets Dad off? But my brother, Mark, who had a newly stitched gut, did not need to be kicked if he arrived first to solve the problem. And what if the police showed up and things got worse and my dad's anger escalated?

The traffic lights changed to red halting those thoughts and a graphic picture from a school project completed years ago careened across my consciousness. My family was obviously Scottish with a last name beginning with Mac. I still recall the project that my brother did in Grade five tracing our family tree. Our deceased mother had stored it in the fragrant cedar chest at the end of my parents' bed for safe keeping. Captain Gillies MacBain, our ancestor from the 18th century, was backed against the wall fighting in the battle of Culloden. His bloodied sword was still swinging in my mind when the traffic light turned green. The image of my family war hero who had killed thirteen men alone before being mortally wounded faded from my mind. Some have horse thieves or famous bank robbers in their heritage but in my heritage are brave men who fought for their families and lands. Gillies lived up to the clan's name on the shield, Touch Not the Cat.

My dad was a roaring lion, and the nurses feared the uncaged cat roaming down the hall kicking doors. This was not a brave or heroic act but one of a crazed man. By the time I arrived, my brother had calmed my dad and the staff had refrained from calling the police. Tranquillizers would be given; the cat would be contained. I returned home to finish out my short night of sleep. That night I dreamed about working in a zoo and when I woke the next day, I mused that I was not just going to a nursing home but to a zoo.

I entered the nursing zoo cautiously that morning. Each occupant was affected differently by disease and their humanity had been exchanged for animal like behaviours. It was almost as if a different, animal-based nature expressed itself through each human occupant. With new eyes, I arrived, not being able to shake the zoo image I had been dreaming about. The parrot-like lady sitting in the wheelchair in the corner of the hall welcomed me with her repeated squawking. "I wanna go home! I wanna go home! I wanna go home!" The nurse would try to quiet her but her piercing bird-like screeches continued to echo through the halls. After passing her, I heard the tall, stooped man softly hooting. He rarely speaks and mostly chants, "Whoo, whoo, whoo." It is like the soft base beat of the nursing home zoo. Another man moves between the tables after the meals picking up all the crumbs off the floor like an anteater grunting gently. Many of the animals are speechless. Their eyes reveal their caged existence as if their human voices have been stolen. One resident paces like a caged tiger going back and forth. Another passes me, the ostrich lady, moving more quickly than the rest. Before I get to my dad's room, I hear the lady who seems to always be crying. Her constant sobbing and moaning remind me of a puppy whimpering for its mother. Exiting my dad's room is a resident monkey thief. Everyone here, at one time or another, steals a banana, a watch, or some trinket from another caged animal, but this woman collects everything not tied down. I have just walked through the zoo exhibit, and I wonder what I will see when I enter my dad's area. There lies my dad sleeping like a gentle giant cat. The snoring is almost purr-like. The MacBain clan shield motto streaks through my mind: Touch Not the Cat. Is it safe now? Which cat will I awaken: the lion or the pussy cat? The human zookeepers are kind and try their best to communicate, to understand, and love the animals, but they must always beware of the angry tiger, the violent gorilla, the howling jackal, or the screeching monkey. I stay longer in the cage today with my dad, but the tranquillized man can barely open his eyes. I see the nature shows in my mind where they lift a huge, tranquillized animal out of a populated area for the safety of the town. He is that animal. I finally wake him up and assist him to sit up. I gently encourage him to stand and lean on his walker. His eyes are glazed with no recognition. No speech can pass his lips. He can barely lift his foot. With a small shuffle, he collapses back down to sit on his bed. Bad behaviour whether violent or sexual often results in this drugged induced state. I lean over and kiss his forehead.

Touch not the cat without a shield. It is the zookeeper's right to safety and the safety of the other caged animals. I get it. I truly do get it. But I don't get it. Is it necessary to drug a man, not an animal but a human, to this level of incapacity? I feel myself making a lamenting keening sound of a grieving baby elephant separated from its parent. I had been through this merry-go-round of Dad's behaviour leading to him being drugged a few times before but never to him being this incapacitated. I and his keepers will ride on it again always trying to balance others' safety while preserving Dad's dignity and safety too. He slumps over and falls back into a drugged, heavy sleep. The visit to the zoo today is finished. I wearily tramp back through the smelly halls, like a baby elephant with sorrow too heavy to carry. Out past the noises, through the stinky pens, and past the locked doors I go. I slump like Dad, but I weep in a corner in my car's cage while he sleeps on in his. There is nothing to say. There is nothing I can do. I return to my home of civility and wonder about my future and the brokenness of it all.

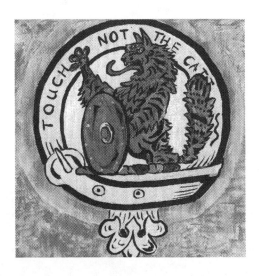

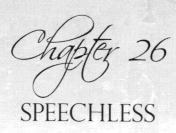

Chapter 26

SPEECHLESS

IF A BOOK ENTITLED <u>How to Increase your Patience through Suffering</u> was published, no one would ever read it. It is unthinkable! Yet suffering, a real part of our existence and this disease can cause patience to grow. Most people, religious or not, have heard of the patience of Job. This man suffered excruciating pain and loss. Physically, his body was riddled with pain and disease. Financially, he experienced huge losses. Emotionally, he suffered through the death of all of his children. And mentally, he was plagued by a whining wife, discouraging friends and his own thoughts. Questions arise when one is suffering. "Why me? This does not benefit anyone, my family or me." We mentally argue. "Why, God?" Even people who give no credence to a God, shake their fist in his imaginary face. Someone must be responsible.

"Why does God not stop it?"

"If He is so good, why do people suffer?"

No one wakes up with the intent to tackle such deep questions but these thoughts haunt throughout the watches of the night for anyone who encounters suffering.

The faces of pain are as varied as the cuts of a diamond. We are multifaceted beings, and our pain can be experienced at differing degrees and in various areas. Even the youngest members of humankind make known their pain through piercing audible sounds.

I was about to earn my first money babysitting as an acne-pocked teenager with steel gray braces. With my backpack in hand, I thought, *"How hard can it be?"* As the father of four parked the family station wagon in front of his suburban home, I, the babysitter, stepped out ready. It would be a short evening of entertaining children and then I would settle into finishing my math module. Three small, blonde Finnish children stood in a row behind their mom who held the fourth child, a three-month-old baby. I took the smallest infant and listened as the mother gave me instructions like a telemarketer not taking a breath. When she finished, I was terrified, but bedtime was only an hour away. I placed the baby in a highchair to watch as the children warmed up slowly to me, their temporary caregiver. Things were going well. The children in pyjamas played duck, duck, goose and hide and seek. Finally, they settled down to listen to an evening bedtime story while eating popcorn. This was a breeze. All three were tucked in and then I turned my attention to the baby with a warmed bottle in hand. Being the youngest I had rarely held or handled a baby. He drank contentedly and I laid him in his crib. That was when the trouble began. He whimpered and then began to cry in full throttle. I picked him up, but he continued his piercing cry.

I couldn't get him to stop so the toddlers scampered from their beds like earwigs under a door demanding, "Make him stop! My mother can, why can't you?"

I began to bounce the baby in my aching arms and the screaming intensified. The children covered their ears.

"We can't go to sleep. You don't know what you are doing! Get our mommy to come home!" They began yelling and crying too.

Panicked, I ran for the phone with the baby in my arms. Father answered. I am sure he could hear the commotion and I could barely think to talk. "Help! What do I do?"

"Put the baby in his crib and leave him there. I'll be right over," Father said firmly with an air of control.

I whisked the child back to his room glad to rid myself of the purple faced, screeching creature. I threw myself on the couch with the crying children. Moments later I heard the thud of a car door as my parents entered the unlocked front door. Mother was wonderful and hugged me, but Father took charge, the man of the hour. All the children stopped and stared as he scooped up the burp cloth and headed for the room where the 747 jet take off crying was escalating.

"There, there," he cooed, picking up the baby and gently thumping his back. A large, strangled burp emerged, accompanied by a runny spit up. The pained baby's shrieking turned to sobs and slowed to heavy heaving and finally whimpers shushed altogether. He patted the baby in rhythm to his off-tune humming. The changed, exhausted and burped baby settled.

"Now off to bed with you. Your brother is fine," my dad directed his comments to the wide-eyed round faces. Like bees to their hive, the children made beelines to their beds. He had settled the house.

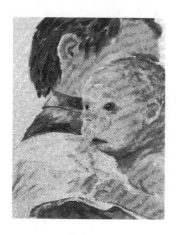

— ❄ —

A time will come for Dad when words will not be able to express needs, pains, or joys. My nana grunted and squawked unintelligible sounds to communicate during the final years of her imprisonment in dementia. I knew she was trapped inside. After awhile, it appeared as though she gave up the struggle and succumbed. Her determined will was washed over and an emptiness in her eyes replaced it, making me wonder if she was even in there anymore.

My dad's speech is losing some flow. Words tumble out of young children. They are fluid in adults but there is a definite loss in a person who is struggling with dementia. It is like a magician is hiding the words in locked boxes and the person is looking for the key to open them. Sometimes I fill in the missing words to keep the conversation going even if we are covering repetitious or nonsensical conversational ground.

Words which are hidden from his mind and repeated partial sentences are the beginnings of speech loss. He may become baby-like with limited means of communication, and I realize that we are beginning to walk down this road together.

Humming familiar songs comforts the inner person who is slowly being shut away because music has the connective power to link you together with the person you are losing. So, I often hum "Jesus loves me. This is know." * A small smile will cross his lips and sometimes I see a clarity pass over his clouding eyes as he looks in my direction. He is assured of Jesus' love for him because as a young man he accepted the forgiveness that Jesus' death provided for him. "For the Bible tells me so"* He has walked and talked with his Saviour for many years. Dad's ultimate hope is in his eternal healing. In heaven Dad will receive a complete healing of mind, body, and soul, even though now he is weak and failing. I finish the song in a triumph but whispered words, "They are weak but He is strong."[13]

---

[13] **Anna Bartlett Warner** (1827–1915)

Chapter 27

FRAGILE HANDLE WITH CARE

BEFORE THE CORONAVIRUS, I WAS DAILY VISITING MY DAD IN THE home. Mary's* piercing sound always screeched through the double locked doors and greeted me with familiarity as I entered the lockdown ward. Hannah* always smiled and mumbled, though I never knew what whispered words she was speaking to me. May* was unpredictable, a wagging finger one day or a coy laugh the next, but I loved her. I would then find my way to the dining hall and see Dad finishing his breakfast or gazing at his plate like a boy not wanting to eat. Since his back was to me, I would always slip up behind him and playfully tickle his shoulder.

"It's me, the food police," I chortled. "How are you?"

The banter is shorter than two years ago when he first came to the nursing home. His hearing has deteriorated, and his conversational skills are diminishing. I would chat it up with the other men at the table and often stay to visit after breakfast. I pull out my paints and canvas as the other residents look on in interest. My dad enjoys just sitting beside me watching me paint some spring or fall scene on the small canvas. It was a new hobby I had taken up to pass time creatively with Dad. He would smile while I was painting and even ask a few limited questions. Often when I finished the scene, he'd say a phrase about what it reminded him of. It was a quiet, but peaceful and reflective time. After packing up my supplies and getting some "oo's" and "ahs" from the staff and other residents, I headed out the way I had come, speaking, and touching the various people I passed.

In the main outer lobby where the more cognitive residents were allowed to roam from their room and even go outside to sit and enjoy the weather, I would often hold the door for some of these residents who used walkers or wheelchairs.

However, today the woman who was following closely behind me was someone I had not met before. "Can you hold the door for me?" she asked.

"Are you sure you can go outside?" I questioned. I looked toward the desk where the administrator usually sat, but she was not there. So, in an error of judgment, I said, "Sure." She wheeled past me, and I walked in the opposite direction to my car. Glancing back over my shoulder, I realized with horror that her wheelchair was careening down the sloped circular driveway heading straight for a curb. My bag of paints and supplies flew up and clattered down to the ground as I leapt over them to intercept that quickly accelerating wheel-chair vehicle. She was two car lengths away. Her waving arms and gray, flying hair were in slowed motion and her scream muffled from the wind, sounded as if she were underwater.

Her helplessness transported me into a childhood memory when I was upside-down under water. My dirty blonde hair was swirling around my face and my hands were waving in the lake water like tentacles, and my scream too, was muffled. I had been hanging on to my father's hand on the cool fall morning, walking along the dock towards a small boat which would take us to a nearby island. My fingers lost his grip when a large, boisterous, woman pushed between us to get to the front of the line. With the connection gone, in my purple fall coat, I toppled headfirst off the dock, unnoticed. Would my father know where I went? Would he glance around? Would he get to me in time?

The lady's screams were asking me the same vital questions? Would I get there in time? Would I catch the racing wheelchair before it slammed into the curb? I ran. I reached. I missed. SLAM. CRASH. THUD. Her body, so fragile was airborne like a broken missile and she landed facedown in the garden past the curb. How could I not have made it? I was so close.

I leaned down, "Are you ok? Stay here," I said stupidly as if she could go anywhere. "I will get help."

The nurses came and hoisted her gently back up into the wheelchair. I had been careless. I should have said, "No". I knew better. Guilt swallowed me up.

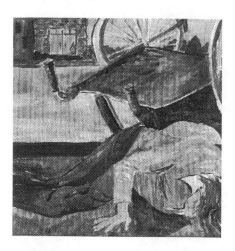

But the woman who had shoved me into the water in her hurried manner did not even look back or know the calamity she had caused. I too, had been thrown and was head- first, down into shallow, sandy water. My father jumped into the cold water to rescue me.

Drenched, he uprighted me and hoisted me out of the water. I was wet, but safe in his arms.

Would she be okay? I deserved the scolding I received from the nurses and was sent on my way. Children are fragile and the elderly even more so. All night I worried about her wellbeing. 'What if she died? It would be all my fault.' The next day, when I came for hymn sing time there sat the lady singing praise to her Lord. Afterward, when I spoke to her, she said, "I only have a scratch, and that is all right." She said coyly, "After all my name is Mrs. Scratch." We both laughed and I smiled. I sent up a grateful prayer to God that she had not been hurt worse.

Elderly folks are fragile, and we must handle them with care. That is a mandate that involves a heart that cares, hands that are gentle, patience that pushes through even when that person is ornery or difficult. But different mandates were about to arrive on the scene.

Chapter 28

I'VE FALLEN AND I CAN'T GET UP

Have you ever seen someone vacuuming, washing windows, and scrubbing the floor with a heavy backpack on? How crazy! Caring for an Alzheimer's loved one is the added backpack in life that you cannot throw off. It weighs down your mind.

Dad enjoyed our regular visits in the nursing home and routines had been established. But one morning, the world was turned upside down. The futuristic horror flick theme we have all watched in movies was rolling out into a new living reality. The year was 2020. All visits from the outside world to the nursing homes were cut off. The perpetrator was not some heinous murderer but a teeny, tiny virus that threatens to undo the world. Its primary target was the elderly, the weakened, and the sickly.

You know the historical question: where were you when JFK was shot or when the twin towers were collapsing? This virus was not a moment in time where you remember exactly where you were but is a mask slowly being pulled over the face of the world. I had kissed my dad on the forehead that particular Saturday morning and told him that my brother would be in later that day. That was the last physical contact I had with him until the government would later change the rules! By the afternoon, I would not be able see him, play the piano for him, or paint beside him. Physically he was fragile, mentally he was collapsing, and now emotionally he would be hurting. Everyday since he had gone into the home, my brother, myself, or my friend, who was almost like a second daughter to him, visited. How would he cope?

These words were blurted over the radio in the car as my heart was slowing from my cardio workout while coming home from the gym. "Nursing homes are now officially closed for visitors. You will not be able to visit until further notice and other measures will be announced as we decide as a nation how to handle this attack."

This was unreal— a 'B' rated movie at best. Really? Words like lockdown, masks, isolation, and social distancing would become the buzz words we would hear as governments in every country decided what tactics they would use to combat the spread of this disease.

Now I felt as though I had dumped my father into some building and abandoned him. He must have felt that too. Nurses, PSW's, and staff all donned masks and everyone looked like puppets with only their eyes visible. All the staff were great, but their faces were now masked. Would the residents think they were in some doctor's soap opera, or would they feel like rats in a lab? His world was upside-down, and he would be drowning in loneliness. Although the outside visitors had been stopped, the workers still moved freely from facility to facility spreading the disease unaware. The government began to get things under control and workers were no longer allowed to work at several different nursing facilities. The overworked health care workers continued to face difficult dilemmas. However, in one nursing home, in another province, it was reported that some elderly folks, who had caught the disease, were gathered in one room, and left alone to die! The public outcry was great! This was worse than imaginable. Thankfully, my dad was in a good facility where the staff were wonderful, but the pressures increased as another staff from other facilities could not substitute in if someone became ill. Staff was often reduced as workers themselves got sick and fewer workers were left to care for residents.

I began to get regular calls. "Your dad has fallen again," and an explanation ensued. Because of mandates we were not allowed in, and my brother and I had committed to walking him daily through the halls, keeping him moving. The busyness of the staff, the decrease of hands-on physical therapy care, and the lack of our presence all played a role in decreasing Dad's mobility. Now Dad was falling more frequently as his strength failed. Then one day the nurse called and told me that Dad was on his way to the hospital, a place that everyone was avoiding like the plague.

"He has fallen, and we think that he has broken his arm or elbow. You will not be able to go the hospital because of the Coronavirus. They will call you and keep you posted." If it were as easy as a jump into the water and uprighting him, like he had done for me so many years ago, I would have taken the plunge, but he had to go it alone, alone to where the diseased gathered. He had no familiar PSW's with him and no family members at his side. There were only masked strangers. Though they were trying to help him, his distraught mind, which was already under siege, would crumble. I hung up the phone and waited for the dreaded call from the hospital. I reflected on his last visit to the hospital: the restraints, the horror, and the craziness. I sat and steeled myself for the call.

With little introduction you could hear the panic and stress in the nurse's voice as she gave me her report. "He is yelling and trying to bite the nurses. We cannot calm him down, even with drugs. We managed to get an x-ray which shows the elbow is broken but laying in a straight line. We cannot even attempt to cast it. He will get hurt or hurt someone in the process. All we can do is to get a sling on him. His heart rate is double, but we will keep him here until his heart rate lowers and then send him back to the nursing home where they will quarantine him."

I knew he would fight. I imagined that he felt like he was in a literal war with the nurses and doctors, and they were the enemy. I have never been a good advocate and I had always left my brother to deal with the nurses and doctors and the drugs they gave him in the home. But the hospital had called me, and I knew that I needed to speak up for Dad. I knew that if they kept him there with an elevated heart rate it would never go down. I sipped in a breath of strengthening air and began my speech. "If you wait for his heart rate to come down you will be dealing with something far greater. He will go into cardiac arrest." I stated firmly. Without taking a breath, I continued, "He will not calm down and if you have done all you can for his arm, then he needs to be immediately sent back to the nursing home before he has a heart attack!"

They heard and were probably just as happy to get the crazed man out of their hospital as fast as possible. The elbow break was aligned, but with a sling which he kept removing. Correct healing would be a challenge. I remember thinking, "*This might be the beginning of the end.*" I had heard from a friend, who was a PSW, that one of her patients fell and broke a bone which led to further falls and more broken bones. I did not want Dad to become Humpy Dumpty and not be able to be put back together because he kept falling off the wall. He was quarantined but watched more closely. It healed slowly. Since the falls out of bed continued, they lowered his bed to a foot from the floor and put a crash pad down to make it more of a roll out of bed than a fall.

In the beginning days of the pandemic, we were only allowed zoom calls which were great for us to see him, but the connection was strained as his eyes darted about. He was unsure about why he could hear and see us, but why we wouldn't come and visit. Explaining that some microscopic germ was marching around the planet infiltrating people and generally targeting the elderly was almost a horror science fiction movie that I found hard to understand, let alone explain it to his failing mind. Our lame attempts to reason with him were exactly that— lame. Different new mandates came from the government which allowed us to make window visits instead of zoom calls. The window visit idea was great, but with a man who is so hard of hearing, these short visits at the window were stressful. For Dad it was like taking him to a donut store. He could see the donut, but he couldn't have one. We were outside, inaccessible, through the glass.

"Just come in," he pleaded on the phone. "I cannot hear what you are saying. How about I come out there?" he continued. Having a conversation was ludicrous.

"What did you have for supper?" I'd ask trying to change the topic.

A confused look crossed his face as he stared down and talked into the phone with a disconnected response. "No, I don't have a puppy."

I would repeat, "What did you have for supper, chicken or fish?"

"No, the dog doesn't have a dish."

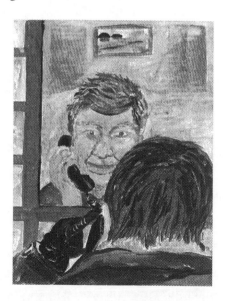

Communication was laughable and heart breaking simultaneously. We would often end up talking to the nurse who was sitting with him and wave at Dad who thought we were by-standers waving at a dignitary. Dad was not himself. Spencer, my middle son, who had carried Dad after he had fallen down the stairs in his home only a few years earlier, stood with me outside the glass and I could see a sense of understanding through Spencer's eyes about the cycle of life. I looked at my son fiddling with his big grown-up hands, and I remember how they were once tiny, baby fingers. They had gripped Grampy's thick, strong hand when Spencer had taken his first and second baby steps. His grandfather, now 20 years later, was weak and fragile and not able to walk much anymore.

Next came the outdoor visits. It was the first time I did not feel like I was visiting an incarcerated prisoner. However, I could not hug or touch him and the six-foot table between my dad continued to challenge meaningful conversation. I was masked and my voice muffled, yet he saw me, recognized me, and smiled, even lifting his broken half healing arm to wave and say "Carolyn".

I finally got used to the daily calls reporting his rolls out of bed. However, the person on the other end of the line that day was not a nurse. The occupational therapist began to explain how I would need to purchase a wheelchair immediately. In Canada, the government helps with the cost. The $5000 wheelchair they deemed necessary, would only cost dad $1200 with subsidies.

My dad was wise with his money and though he did have enough to cover this cost, I knew my dad. He never paid full price for anything, and he wouldn't want us too either. When my father was purchasing my mother's casket, he tried to make a deal with the undertaker suggesting a two for one deal. He would want my brother and I to at least try to find a deal. Wheelchair shopping though, is not like shopping for groceries where you can use coupons or price match. There are size constraints of the knee to floor, backrest width and seat depth dimensions all which need to be met.

I began my search by calling two people, who I knew had been through this recently, to ask for suggestions. I found one on Facebook marketplace for $650. It had all the right dimensions except it was 16 inches wide not the 20-inch width I needed. I made my husband stand at attention while I measured his hips. Did 4 inches to sit your bottom in a chair really mean that much? I concluded it did. I crossed that one off the list of possibilities. Then one friend, whom I had contacted, but lived in the next county, informed me that she had found an almost perfect wheelchair about an hour away from London. It was a God provision because I would never have looked in that area. The width of the chair was 2 inches wider than needed and the knee to foot measurement was one inch shorter. We drove out to meet the sellers of the bright blue, impeccable chair. When you meet people who have gone through the same ordeal, there is an instant connection. You exchange stories of sadness and together there is a shared burden of understanding. The people selling the chair had a mother with Alzheimer's who had only used it for a year and a half. They graciously allowed us to inspect the chair to see if the height of the chair could be adjusted through raising the wheels and the footrest could be lowered. They gave us a great price! We got the deal! Dad would be so proud and the folks selling it were thrilled that someone else could make use of it.

As we drove away with the wheelchair in the back of the truck it was bittersweet. Driving was my dad's passion. He drove the city bus with pizzazz down the streets of London, but now he'd be meandering with a wheelchair down the halls of the nursing home. From riding in a baby buggy, to crawling, to walking, to running, to shuffling, and finally back in a buggy, a bright blue wheelchair, was sad. The only bright side to this was knowing that he will run again. He will run into the arms of His Saviour in Heaven next.

Chapter 29

YOU CAN'T DUCK DEATH

WE'D ALL ADJUSTED TO THE CORONAVIRUS AND WITH REGULAR nose swabs and appropriate masking we were allowed to resume visits as before. One day as I was coming in for a visit, I found the nurse struggling to rebuild the broken leg of the piano keyboard stand which my dad had kicked in frustration just moments before my arrival. I felt broken too as I took over and collapsed the legs of the broken stand. Humbling myself I sat crossed legged on the floor where I had placed the keyboard to play hymns on it one last time for Dad. Even with my mask on, stifling my voice, I sang as loud as I could. It calmed him and as always, the words of the great old songs challenged my heart to keep going too. It was time to remove the piano. It was broken and it needed to be retired or repaired. I tapped his shoulder goodbye and headed to the door with all the pieces and parts of the broken keyboard. Since the load was awkward, I stumbled out through his room door and had to set everything down. Even though I had walked out of his bedroom door hundreds of times in the last few years, I had never noticed the plaque that hung in that corridor just above my jumbled mess. It was as if God was reaching through the clouds and speaking directly to my downcast heart: The words on the plaque were poignant: *Disappointments are God's way of saying, I've got something better in mind*! Wow, even when you want to be angry, give up, yell, or have a hissy fit, God says, "I've got this! Trust me!"

Death was on the horizon for Dad, but only God decides his ending date. The moment one sucks in one's first breath of air in a hospital delivery room the countdown begins for all of us. We live in denial. Women use creams and make-up to falsely extend the look of youth. Men lift weights. Beauty equals youth, youth equals life, but in reality, the body is decaying.

Many Wednesday nights after prayer meeting during my growing up years, we stopped into funeral homes for visitations. People we knew like Martha*, the lady who always wore the green hat, or Joe*, the older gentlemen who usually carried candy in his pockets for the kids could be viewed. These old people lay in beautiful wooden boxes while everyone walked by. My brothers and I followed our parents like ducks down the stream paddling through the solemn halls of the funeral parlours. It was like a wax museum for me. I knew these acquaintances, but until death steals a person one loves, only then, does the reality of it knock one flat.

Cancer eats, gnaws, and destroys your physical body piece by piece. The medical answer is to poison with chemo, burn using radiation, or cut to remove tumours, yet the monster, the return of the "C" word, always lurks in the shadows. Death by cancer is brutal. I heard my mother's bones break with every hug or movement on the bed, yet she refused to take more morphine than absolutely necessary. My stepmother drowned with her lungs filling slowly in her fight with cancer.

My papa died of a heart attack clutching the partially built chain link fence while gripping his chest because a piece of plaque lodged in the blood pathway to his heart. Cholesterol, tiny bits of fat, made it difficult for blood to squeeze through veins, and on that day the path blocked fully, blood backed up and seeped out in all directions looking, but finding no alternate path. Time was short. Pain was intense. Life ebbed away.

Dementia is not as time conscious, although some days I wish it were. I do not remember the day Nana died, just that it was sad. But in some ways, it was a relief for my parents. The journey for the person riddled with dementia and the caregiver alike is extremely difficult. For the patient their physical body slows but is mostly left in tack until the very end stages. For the caregiver, the mental mind of the person you know dies in stages right before your eyes. Although the future may provide ways to shorten the process through euthanasia, this is only a short cut to the same reality, death. Pain, suffering, and grief must be lived, felt, and shared because the long-drawn-out death of a loved one may be necessary for restitution, forgiveness, or other reasons that we cannot fathom or understand until many years pass.

There is some dignity however, in dying with your mind intact. My mother wrote, leaving for each of us treasured letters to look back upon. Those who have heart attacks leave current memories with their spouses and grandchildren to rehearse and reflect upon. However, diseases of the mind steal the person of sensibility and rob the family of their good memories. Both experience nonsense, stress, and loneliness.

A few years ago, we came close to losing Dad to a heart attack. During the visit with the heart specialist, he prescribed a medicine, but explained that we probably needed to stop his other medication for the dementia as they would interfere with one another. After a month on the new meds, my brother and I did notice significant changes for the worse, mentally. Had we made the wrong decision about which pills to give Dad, the pink ones not the yellow ones? I felt like I was living in the surreal world of the Wizard of Oz. Could these medicines give my dad the heart that Tin Man desired, or get a brain that Scarecrow wanted? I know what I would want, a mind in tack and to die of a heart attack. Could my dad even make such a choice for himself? In frustration I decided to tell Dad what each pill could do as I pulled out the yellow ones down from the cupboard which Mark was no longer giving him. "Dad, these pills used to help you to be more with it and not as forgetful, less agitated, while these pink pills help your heart to function properly," I explained as I held up each bottle of magic pills. Of course, using his diminishing brain capacity, he does not think that he forgets and totally denies that he gets agitated, so for a while we continue with the heart choice and the dementia worsens. Finally, my brother and I would make the switch choosing the brain over the heart. It was kind of like going hunting, something was going to die.

My brother and my father enjoyed hunting together. Often it was more about tramping through the woods on chilly fall days because big game like deer eluded them. Shooting clay pigeons at the outdoor gun club was great practice for hunting birds. Donning their orange coats and gear they headed out on adventures. Many times they hunkered down but they missed the targets as the ducks rose up over the open water and flew safely out of range. Maybe it was due to not having a hunting dog, poor aim, or a soft spot in dad's heart for ducks, but I don't recall ever having duck for dinner. They did mange to shoot a few partridges over the years and we enjoyed them at meals.

My dad was no longer the hunter but the hunted. Death was stalking him. In the nursing home they took over the medications balancing the choice between brain and heart. These were now left up to new doctors. Yet it felt like he was dying slowly on both fronts: the heart and the brain. His physical mobility was also gone. I felt the squeeze of the smallness of his world, but there was a bright spot that surprised me. Driving to the nursing home for almost four years, several days a week, I noticed, as though for the first time, the duck pond not a kilometer away. My brain shot into full gear. I would push the wheelchair through the suburb and talk to him while passing through the chain linked walkway that bridged the neighborhood suburb to the natural wildlife park. We loved that spring because the mother ducks waddled with their baby ducklings all around the base of his parked wheelchair. Their fuzzy yellow feathers and cute little parades brought such smiles to the aged man and me. This place became our haven of refuge. Small delights of joy can be found if one seeks out these moments. Spring morphed into summer and the ducks glided into the pond unafraid of the once great hunter. Dad loved to feed them and nodded at the moms and children who strolled through on their walks to see the ducks too. Coming here was like watching a big screen TV of the outdoors.

However, the warm comfortable sun of summer was losing its heat and turning into the next season. The last day in fall, I bundled him up in his coat and blanket and we headed to the pond, but it felt different. A chill was in the air. The breeze had a cold scent of death, but I pressed on to our piece of heaven. The ducks were there as always, but after I had locked the wheels of his chariot, I looked up and saw something on the horizon through the fog. A flock of Canadian geese blackened the sky! Hoards of them and they seemed headed our way. The ducks quickly waddled away from us and back to their pond to wait and see if the black cloud was going to pass them by or crowd them in. Honk! Honk! They noisily splashed down and skidded in. The ducks were feeling pushed out so they in unison took flight upward in the opposite direction. The big dark aggressive geese settled in like a portent of the coming winter of my dad's life. Death was coming.

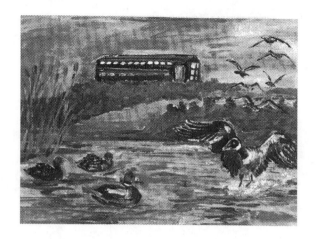

Chapter 30

THE FINAL CURTAIN

A TEAR SLIPPED UNDER MY MASK AND ALMOST PLOPPED ON THE sympathy card that lay below the framed picture at the nursing home. I stood in shock as I signed my condolences for Mike*, the old Chinese man, who had a wonderful smile. Many of the residents I had gotten to know over the last few years were passing away. Some died from loneliness, some from refusing to eat, some from old age, and others from a myriad of other reasons. As I turned away, there was his daughter holding the door for the maintenance man wheeling her father's few belongings out: a chair, a fan, a tv, a book, and a few used boxes of puzzles. My eyes naturally looked down because it seemed like a premonition of the journey I would be walking soon. A lone puzzle piece on the floor caught my attention. I was about to call out to the daughter when the door clicked shut. I stood holding a small piece of the puzzle in my hands. He was gone. The puzzle of his life was complete from life to death.

My dad was a survivor moving into the second year of a worldwide pandemic in a nursing home. My brother and I were to be locked out of his life again. We were his essential caregivers, who were not only visiting him, wheeling him about, but helping in the feeding process too. It was a challenge like feeding a toddler! However, when he eyed the treats that we brought in, he would often eat for the reward. Through angry tears my brother wagged his finger at the nursing home staff predicting, "If you follow these mandates and deny us access, my dad will be dead in three weeks!" We knew his life depended upon our assistance. They were in a difficult spot, and like most places of business, they obeyed the demands of the government.

During that first week dad barely consumed anything. We knew because we got a call that his urine was discoloured; we guessed he was going septic. The stress pressed in, and we didn't know what to do. Would he starve to death and die alone thinking his children didn't care about him any longer? Into the second week we were informed that Covid had crept into the building again through the vaccinated workers and now the residents would be locked into their rooms to keep it at bay. A few days later we got yet another call that he'd contracted the virus in his weakened state.

After not being allowed in for two full weeks, we received our final call. My knees buckled as I stood in the fitness store hanging on to dumbbells, not because of the weight of the physical bells, but because of the weighted phone call. "Your father is palliative," the nurse on the other end stated flatly.

The pain pierced my heart. He was fine two weeks ago and yet it was an answer to a prayer, an unwelcome answer. I had asked that God would open my dad's eyes to see an angelic companion in his room since he was completely alone in his room, and we could not visit. Now we were being called to come back in as essential caregivers because he was officially dying. We would be the presence I had prayed for, a physical mortal presence, until he would see the angels in Heaven and Jesus, His Saviour, who would welcome him in. What an amazing but terrifying, and seemingly cruel answer to my prayer! I was crushed!

I quickly drove up to the nursing home that had housed him for so long and proceeded to don the clothing of a biohazard worker. But I would not be treating my beloved dad as a specimen. I reached out and hugged him and stepped back to momentarily lift my mask so he could know it was me. There sat the shell of the man I loved, and it took everything in me to hold back the dam of tears that threatened to breach my watering eyes. During the next six days my brother and I held his hands, rubbed his feet, stroked his back, sang to him, and whispered that we loved him. There was one very precious moment when we heard his almost inaudible, slurred response, "I uv you too".

We were not there the moment death swept in that cold, January, Sunday morning when his breathing finally stopped. Arriving shortly after, my brother and I wept, prayed, and hugged one another in that claustrophobic room that had housed him for his last years. My emotions swelled. I was numb. The pain, the grief, the weight, and the ache threatened to swallow me up.

My mind was flooded with so many things. But my dad's favourite portion of scripture, Psalm 100, rose to the top. *"Make a joyful noise unto the Lord, . . . come before his presence with singing. . . and may God's faithfulness continue to all generations."*[14] My dad had no ability to sing a note on tune. Instead, he made a joyful noise, singing on his bus routes through the streets of London to cheer his passengers for many years. Yet, somehow, his grandchildren received the gift of music. Two of my sons were leading worship music in our church service while my brother and I were saying our goodbyes to the body of Lyndon, empty of his spirit laying on the bed. Although we didn't see his passing, his body was still warm, and his lips were beginning to blue in a slightly opened position. As I looked upon my dad, for the final time, I imagined him singing in perfect pitch his favourite song <u>Heavenly Sunshine</u> in the very throne room of God. We left to go to Sunday service at Dad's church, the one I'd grown up in which was near the nursing home. As we walked in, they were singing a lively version of <u>When we all get to Heaven</u>. It was hard

---

[14]   Psalm 100:1,2,5 King James Version

to hold my quivering body and reddening eyes from revealing fresh grief. Though my heart's melody was one of lament, tears flushed into joy for him at the realization his pain was over. Through Jesus he had only tasted death but now was in the presence of his Saviour. His life had ended here, and the earthly fog forever lifted, and rays of eternity engulfed him.

Now it was time for the funeral. It surprised me, although it shouldn't have, when one of the staff members at the funeral parlor commented to me that she knew my dad from taking his bus years ago. Wow! The lives he had touched, and his influence did not seem to end. Even the person dressing his body for the casket knew him!

Planning the funeral, even though most of it was paid for in advance, was still chaotic. I almost missed putting some names in the obituary and to make matters worse, I arranged the funeral on my brother's birthday and then had to change all the plans. It was tumultuous! No time for grief or reflection.

By Wednesday, I was ready to go back into the nursing home to clear out his things, or so I thought. At the front door they asked me if I had brought boxes to pack up his belongings. I realized that I wasn't thinking clearly because what should have been obvious wasn't. I was still in that fog that had lasted for almost eight years. So, after being directed, I went behind the nursing home and began to dig through the dumpster of cardboard and pull out several brown boxes. The cold stung my fingers and I felt like a homeless person scrounging through garbage. By the time I dragged all the boxes down the hall and sat in his room on the floor I felt the rush of a January thaw swirling over me. Death was frigid in the room just a few days before, but this new wave of grief was messy and wet, and I bawled! The nurses and helpers had already bagged some of his clothes. Vicky*, an occupational therapist in the unit, slipped into the room and helped me sort through the books, DVDs, and the other odds and ends. After she left, I was alone again staring at the huge cart stacked with six garage bags of clothes and seven boxes of things. I collapsed! "But God didn't I pray that you would orchestrate the timing and manner of his death to bring You the most glory," I whispered and struggled in my thoughts. I looked out through the window into the courtyard, empty of living plants or life, and figured this prayer was unanswered.

But quietly, in my spirit, My Heavenly Father whispered to my heart, *"My child, don't you see? You couldn't even plan his funeral for this Saturday, the convenient day to bury him, because even his belongings are My final act of service I will use from his life".* My heart leapt as I realized that the difficulty in finding a burial date because of a fund-raising event and my brother's birthday had a reason. We settled on a funeral date, almost two weeks out, because God wanted me to collect the last things this man had on earth and add it to the collection for the fund raiser ending that Saturday. The monies would be used for orphans and widows in Ukraine before his body would be committed to the ground.

I imagined my dad smiling and saying, "Great timing! I don't need those things anymore." At that moment, I recognized that even the timing of his death was part of God's calendar of purpose, and it warmed my heart.

"The glory is truly yours, God." I rose and walked out of the nursing home and the fog lifted.

Chapter 31

EPILOGUE

I WOULD BE REMISS IF I DID NOT INCLUDE MY FATHER'S SPIRITUAL journey to God. His passion was to share Christ with everyone he met. He met my mother after he moved from Nova Scotia to Toronto. She had accepted Jesus as her Saviour and was concerned to date someone who did not believe or know her God. She brought him to church to hear about Jesus. The man behind the pulpit talked of how the world was created perfect by a loving God. He spoke of Adam and Eve and their choice to disobey God plunging all people into a broken world. Their choice brought death, disease, and separation between God and people. Dad's hands clenched the pew in front of him as the man continued explaining that God loved the world of people so much that he sent Jesus to come to earth. Dad had relayed this story to me so often about how he felt the preacher was talking directly to him about how the innocent Son of God would die in his place for the things that he had done wrong. My dad began to understand. He knew he was far from perfect and not deserving of this kind of love, yet he wanted it.

"If you believe and trust that Jesus' death cover's your guilt and sin, you will be saved," the man proclaimed from the pulpit' and in that moment, Lyndon chose to believe. He understood the depth of

God's love for him and he began a spiritual journey with the Lord that spanned his life and carried him into the next world.

"Precious in the sight of the Lord are the death of his saints."[15]

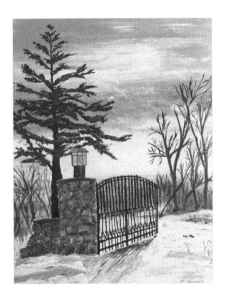

---

[15]   Psalms 116:15 King James Version.

Author's Note

As a new artist and writer, I thank my husband, John, for encouraging me to write down my feelings and thoughts for this memoir. I also want to thank you for taking the journey through the fog with Lyndon and his family. If you want to reach out to me, I would love to hear from you. Email me at:

bagnallcarolyn@hotmail.com
I also have an art website and a children's book website as well:
artworkscarolyn.com
mrsbbookroom.com
God Bless.

Printed in the United States
by Baker & Taylor Publisher Services